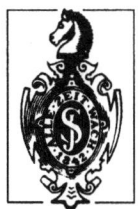

A. E. Baranov · D. Densow
T. M. Fliedner · H. Kindler

Clinical Pre Computer Proforma for the

International Computer Database for Radiation Exposure Case Histories

Edited by the WHO-Collaborating Centre
for Radiation Emergency Medical Preparedness and Assistance
(CREMPA) at the Institute of Occupational Medicine,
University of Ulm, Germany

Springer-Verlag
Berlin Heidelberg New York London Paris
Tokyo Hong Kong Barcelona Budapest

Prof. Dr. Alexander Baranov
Ministry of Health
of the Russian Federation
Institute of Biophysics
Marshall Novikov Street 23
123098 Moscow, Russia

Dr. med. Dirk Densow
Prof. Dr. med. Dr. h.c. T. M. Fliedner
Dipl.-Inform. Med. Hauke Kindler

Institut für Arbeits- und Sozialmedizin
University of Ulm
Albert-Einstein-Allee 11
89081 Ulm, Germany

ISBN-13:978-3-540-57596-2   e-ISBN-13:978-3-642-78740-9
DOI: 10.1007/978-3-642-78740-9

The use of general descriptive names, registered names, trademarks, etc. in this publication does not imply, even in the absence of a specific statement, that such names are exempt from the relevant protective laws and regulations and therefore free for general use.

Product liability: The publishers cannot guarantee the accuracy of any information about dosage and application contained in this book. In every individual case the user must check such information by consulting the relevant literature.

Typesetting: Camera ready copy from the author/editor

21/3130 - 5 4 3 2 1 0 - Printed on acid-free paper

FOREWORD

This publication provides guidance on preparing data to be input into an international computerised database for clinical case histories of persons accidentally exposed to whole body irradiation. The publication has resulted from a close collaboration between the Institute of Biophysics including its Hospital Number 6 in Moscow, Russia, and the Institute of Occupational and Social Medicine at the University of Ulm. In both institutions, much experience has been accumulated during the last 20 years in dealing with basic and clinical research in the field of radiation accident management. In both institutions many case histories of radiation accident victims have been recorded. On this basis the scientists and clinicians from both institutions developed, over the last two years, a pre computer proforma to feed the International Computer Database for Radiation Exposure Case Histories, with standardised data from clinical case histories of radiation accident victims.

This activity should be seen as part of WHO efforts to establish a network of institutions around the world, competent in Radiation Emergency Medical Preparedness and Assistance. This network has become known as REMPAN and it is prepared to provide medical advice and assistance when a radiation accident occurs in any country. The Institute of Occupational and Social Medicine, at the University of Ulm, is part of this global network.

The establishment of the computerised database for radiation accident clinical case histories is a major step in the development of a computerised guide for physicians who might have to deal in the future with the diagnosis and treatment of overexposed persons, following a radiation accident.

The international database to be established may be used by all member states of the World Health Organisation and other countries in which radiation accidents have occurred or might occur in the future.

Dr. I. Riaboukhine
Radiation Scientist
Division of Environmental Health
World Health Organisation, Geneva

PREFACE

In April 1990, the Ministry of Health of the Russian Federation, through the Institute of Biophysics in Moscow, and the University of Ulm, Institute of Occupational and Social Medicine, agreed to jointly develop an International Radiation Accident Database for Case Histories to record the acute medical consequences in persons accidentally exposed to ionising radiation.

In order to establish such an international database, it became necessary in the first step to harmonise the reporting and recording of all clinical signs and symptoms observed in accidentally exposed persons. In the Institute of Biophysics, more than 500 persons suffering from consequences of acute radiation exposure have been clinically observed. In the Institute of Occupational and Social Medicine of the University of Ulm an attempt has also been made to record clinical signs and symptoms of persons as reported in the scientific medical literature.

As a consequence of this collaborative effort between the institutes in Moscow and Ulm, the Pre Computer Proforma was developed to help the physicians record patient data in a unified and standardised fashion in order to allow for the establishment of the International Computer Database for Radiation Exposure Case Histories (MURAD). The purpose of MURAD is to bring together in one computerised database – by means of international scientific co-operation – as many clinical case histories of the acute radiation syndrome as possible. In scientific literature it is not usually possible to review the individual clinical course in a day-to-day analysis. The availability of access to a case-oriented database, however, seems to be desirable for several reasons:

- support of medical research on the acute radiation syndrome,
- decision support by providing case histories for comparison,
- development of medical management strategies,
- evaluation and development of grading schemes for the acute radiation syndrome,
- evaluation of a computerised guide for physicians to help deal with radiation injuries,
- test of predictive simulation models of haematopoiesis,
- support medical education as a source of exemplary case histories, and
- give access to relevant data for the international scientific community.

The authors are pleased to present this Pre Computer Proforma to the scientific community for general use. During a conference held in Ulm in December 1992 which brought together the 8 WHO Collaborating Centres on Radiation Emergency Medical Preparedness and Assistance – REMPAN, the present Pre Computer Proforma was presented, extensively discussed, and recommended for use in the scientific community.

This Clinical Pre Computer Proforma is to be used for the recording of patient data for the International Computer Database for Radiation Exposure Case Histories. Thereby, it is hoped that the scientific community will have at their disposal information on clinical observations made in the course of the treatment of acute radiation accident victims. This database will thus be an important basis for research and development in the field of medical radiation protection actions, aiming to improve existing, and develop new approaches in the treatment of radiation accident victims. This goal will be supported by the development of a computerised guide for physicians treating radiation injuries in human beings. This work is presently in progress in both institutions.

This, however, will only be possible if you return your filled-in copy to the addressees named in the introduction.

Acknowledgement

The authors acknowledge the continuous encouragement and support of the following institutions: the Environmental Health Division of the World Health Organisation; the Commission of the European Communities, the Federal Ministry of Health of the Federal Republic of Germany; the Ministry of Science and Research of the State of Baden-Württemberg; and the University of Ulm.

Moreso, we gratefully appreciate the scientific advice provided to us by a number of scientists and radiation protection physicians: Dr. E. P. Cronkite, Brookhaven National Laboratories, Brookhaven, NY; Prof. Dr. A. K. Guskova, Medical Director of the Hospital No. 6, Moscow; Academician Prof. Dr. L. A. Ilyin, Director of the Institute of Biophysics, Moscow; Dr. R. C. Ricks, Director of Oak Ridge Institute of Science and Education, Oak Ridge, TN; and Prof. Dr. T. Szepesi, Radiology Department of the Allgemeines Krankenhaus, Vienna.

In addition, our work has been made possible by the indefatigable help of our associates, graduate students, and our competent secretarial staff.

We wish to thank also Dr. U. Heilmann of the Springer Publishing Company who by her advice allowed for the publication of the questionnaire in its present form.

The authors

Introduction to the Use of the Pre Computer Proforma

Introduction to the Use of the Pre Computer Proforma

Welcome to this questionnaire! The Institute of Occupational Health, WHO Collaborating Centre for Radiation Emergency Medical Preparedness and Assistance at the University of Ulm and the Institute of Biophysics, Ministry of Health of the Russian Federation, as authors of this Clinical Pre Computer Proforma greatly appreciate your participation in this joint research effort to build up an International Computer Database for Radiation Exposure Case Histories.

This scientific endeavour is dedicated to the improvement of the knowledge on the acute radiation syndrome which is in fact a rare disease. Consequently, it is worthwhile to collect all accessible case histories. We acknowledge your effort in accompanying us on our way towards this goal. Since English has become the language generally accepted throughout the scientific community we kindly request that you fill in this questionnaire in English.

A case will be eligible for the International Computer Database for Radiation Exposure Case Histories if the patient has been involved in a radiation accident with subsequent exposure to ionising radiation.

We did not decide to fix a certain threshold dose as a criterion for inclusion as a case in the database. Initially, we ask you to submit data about the acute period. The length of this period is defined by the following clinical conditions:

- the time of recovery from the post-irradiation myelodepression (usually not more then 4 months after acute irradiation, and possibly longer, after the end of protracted or chronic over-exposure) or

- the time of death from causes related to the acute radiation syndrome.

Your remarks on both the content and form of this questionnaire are welcome. Feel free to call on us if any questions arise or to express your approval or disapproval. Please use either address as return address for your completed proforma

Prof. Dr. Alexander Baranov, M. D.
Clinical Hospital No 6
Marshal Novikov Street 23
123098 Moscow
Russian Federation
tel: 007/095/1904591
fax: same as tel
email alex@baranov.msk.SU

Prof. Dr. T. M. Fliedner, M. D.
Institute of Occupational and Social Medicine
University of Ulm
Albert-Einstein-Allee 11
D-89081 Ulm
FR Germany
tel:+731/502-34 00, fax: +731/502 3415
email kindler@dulfaw1a.bitnet

In most cases you will find the questionnaire self explanatory. However, in some cases there may be doubt as to the best way to enter the data. The necessary information is given below.

One typical design feature of this questionnaire is its hierarchical structure both as far as the order of the organ systems is concerned (see Table of Contents) but also reflecting the order and structure of the items you are asked for.

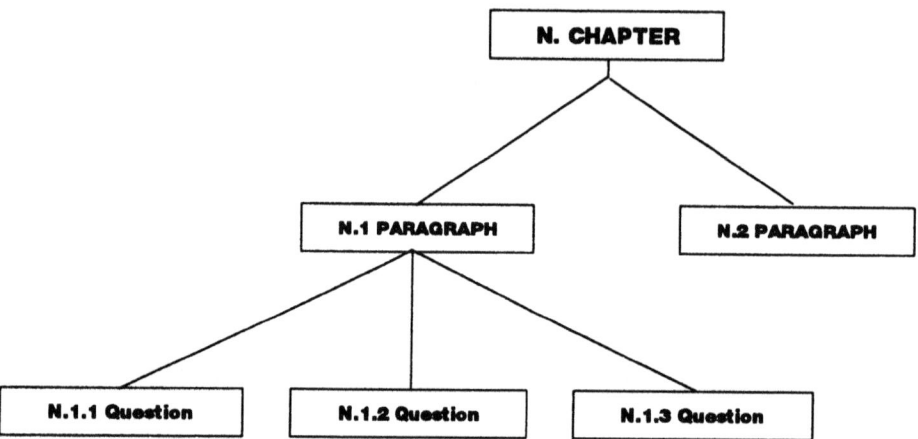

Fig. 1 - Hierarchical structure of the questionnaire.

Each chapter (one digit), paragraph (two digits separated by a period), and question (three digits separated by periods) is introduced by a headline which is also related to the table of contents.

3.1.1   Dyspeptic Symptoms and Enlargement of Parotid Glands

The second line starts with a group of check boxes. They serve to identify whether one or more items as defined subsequently have occurred in the patient.

all no ☐, all unknown ☐

if this is true for one of the items, the line should read:

all no ☒, all unknown ☐

Each time you indicate "all no" or "all unknown" the subsequent part of the questionnaire must not contain any entries. If you identify facts as unknown you may instead of indicating "uk" leave the check box empty as well as the rest of the corresponding line.

The headline and the check boxes are then followed by the different types of questions. The following examples illustrate the typical data formats you will encounter.

Typical Data Format

1.   Free Text
The simplest way to enter the data is free text. In these tables you are allowed to enter as much text as necessary.

family name	*Miller*

Fig. 2   Table to enter free text

2.   Check Boxes
These tables provide at least two alternatives from which to choose. Indicate by placing a "☒" in the appropriate box.

sex	male ☒	female ☐

Fig. 3   Table with check boxes

3.   Numerical Entries
The required format of the data to be entered in this type of table is numerical. The appropriate dimension or order of magnitude can be identified either in the headline or elsewhere close to the enter box

age at the time of the accident [yy]	46	date of birth [dd.mm.yyyy]	10.04.1947

Fig. 4   Table for numerical entries

All of the tables are constructed from these three elements appearing either in combination or alone, in either horizontal or vertical order.

The following exemplary tables demonstrate the most important types of data.

Typical Data Tables

Clinical signs and symptoms are recorded in table form. See fig. 5. Table space is provided for the entry of free text (below nausea and vomiting) in case you wish to enter another or a repetitively occurring symptom or sign. You will find check boxes to indicate whether a particular symptom or sign has occurred. Finally, you have boxes to enter numerical data for onset, end, maximum, and degree of the respective sign or symptom. Repetitive occurrence of the disorders must be described separately (see "nausea" in fig. 8 of this manual). For that purpose use either an empty row (as shown below) or copy one empty table from Annex 8.7 and attach it to the corresponding table. Do not cross out items on the lists and replace them with other entries.

Since we consider temporal aspects to be of vital importance for a true case–to–case comparison we have devoted a chapter of this manual (see below) to the usage of time. The system by which we code the severity is outlined directly after this exemplary table.

Symptom	yes	no	uk	Begin (Date & Time)	End (Date & Time)	Maximum (Date & Time)	Degree
nausea	☒	☐	☐	12.08.1993	16.08.1993	14.08.1993	2
vomiting	☐	☒	☐				
diarrhoea	☒	☐	☐	12.08.1993	16.08.1993	14.08.1993	2

Fig. 5   Clinical signs and symptoms table

Grading

For the grading of clinical signs and symptoms a five grade ordinary scale should be used. The five degrees are as follows:

1	mild
2	moderate
3	severe
4	very severe
5	fatal

The second type of table is intended for the recording of numerical data. To enter date and time when required you should follow the rules as outlined below. If at all possible, please be sure to use date and time of sampling. The laboratory values should, if appropriate, be entered as numerical values with or without conversion to SI - units. Fractions or multiples should be expressed in exponential form. In order to proceed with the conversion properly please refer to paragraphs 8.2 and 8.3. You are also requested to give the normal range of your laboratory parameters in table 8.6. If you do not use SI units please state this fact clearly in the table.

	Date and Time	RBC [Tera/l]	Haemo-globin [g/l]	Haema-tocrit [%]	MCV [femto-l]	Reticulo-cytes [%]	Platelets [Giga/l]	ESR [mm/h]	WBC [Giga/l]
1	12.08.1993 15:00	5.6	15.5	46	90	0.5	250	25	8
2	12.08.1993 20:00		15.6			0.7			12
3	13.08.1993 06:00		15.3			0.3	280		10

Fig. 6   Numerical data table

Another type of table serves to record the antibiogramms. To enter date and time where required, you should follow the rules as outlined below. The multiple (or the fraction) should be expressed in exponential form (see paragraph 8.3, e.g., 1 Tera/l = 1e12/l). Please note that all listed drugs should be recorded using International Non Proprietary Names (INN). If further information on INN is required please refer to chapter 4.4. Be sure to always use the same order of tested drugs to allow for easier filling–in of several tables.

Date and Time	16.08.1993 03:15	16.08.93 06:00	16.08.93 09:00	
Source of Material	blood	urine	blood	
Species	pseudomonas aeruginosa	e. coli	pseudomonas aeruginosa	
No. of Microbes per g or ml of Material	1e6	1e6	54e6	
Drugs :				
1 Azlocillin	+	uk	0	
2 Carbenicillin	-	uk	-	
3 Cefotaxim	0	+	0	
4 Polymyxin B	0	uk	-	
5 Cefazolin	uk	+	uk	
6 Mezlocillin	uk	0	uk	
7 Gentamycin	uk	+	uk	
8				

Fig. 7   Antibiogramm table

Usage of Time

As stated above, temporal aspects are very important. Therefore, all entries should be labelled with a set of time parameters. In order to avoid inconvenience to the potential user of our pre computer proforma several time formats will be acceptable.

The following example provides you with the necessary details. Let us assume for exemplary reasons that an accident occurred on the 12th of August at 1:00 p.m.. Accordingly, the entries will read:

Symptom	yes	no	uk	Begin (Date & Time)	End (Date & Time)	Maximum (Date & Time)	Degree
nausea	☒	☐	☐	*1h2m*	*2d 06:56*	*1d 23:04*	*3*
vomiting	☐	☒	☐				
nausea	☒	☐	☐	*15.08.1993 14:02*	*18.08.1993 06:56*	*16.08.1993 03:08*	*2*

Fig. 8   Clinical signs and symptoms table showing all possible usages of time

The table indicates that the patient felt nauseated starting from the 12th of August 1993 2:02 p. m. Nausea persisted until the 13th of August at 6:56 a. m. with a maximum of 3 (severe nausea) at around midnight. Nausea relapsed August 15 through 18, with a maximum on August 16, 1993. However, the patient did not experience vomiting.

If, on the other hand, you prefer to give date and time as relative to the date and time of the accident, you are also welcome to do so. In principle 3 time formats are appropriate:

Begin (Date & Time)	syntax	Description	Comments
1h12m	(number)h (number)m	relative time	during the first 24 hours after the exposure
1d 06:35	(number)d (time) in 24hour format	relative date + astronomic time	
14.08.93 14:00	day and month as two digits, time 24hour format	calendar date + astronomic time, years with two digits	
14.08.1993 14:00	day and month as two digits, time 24hour format	calendar date + astronomic time, years with four digits	this format is preferred, the database will contain all data in this form

Fig. 9   Time formats allowed

Time granularity

If you are able to give temporal data, i. e. date and time in the formats as laid out above, time granularity, the minimal distance between two points of time, will be one minute. If you do not give the minutes the granularity will be restricted to one hour. If both hours and minutes are not known the granularity will further be reduced to one day. the following table sums this up and relates temporal data and time granularity. In addition to the information on the granularity this table also gives you the necessary details on how to fill in temporal data if you lack exact temporal information.

point of time	astronomic date and time	relative time	granularity
exact date and time known	14.08.1993 14:24	1d0h0m	1 minute
date known exactly, time: only hours are known	14.08.1993 15	1d0h	1 hour
only date is known	15.08.1993	1d	1 day
only month is known	09.1993		1 month
only year is known	1994		1 year

Fig. 10   Obtainable time granularity

If the site of the accident and the site of treatment lie in different time zones, all temporal data should be entered in the time zone of the treatment in preference to the time zone of the accident. This is sensible since a larger amount of data is normally acquired at the place of treatment. Please indicate in the accident description that there is a time difference.

Relative temporal data must refer to the beginning of the radiation exposure. If the latter is unknown, you are requested to refrain from using relative temporal data.

Distinction between onset and observation

Please enter the data, e.g., date and time, when clinical signs and symptoms first occur. However, if that is for some reason impossible, one may indicate when these signs and symptoms were first observed. This is expressed by using a "?" in front of the date.

Symptom	yes	no	uk	Begin (Date & Time)	End (Date & Time)	Maximum (Date & Time)	Degree
nausea	☒	☐	☐	?12.08.1993	16.08.1993	14.08.1993	2

Fig. 11   Clinical signs and symptoms table when for the beginning of a symptom, only the date of first observation is known

Consequently, the line above reads that the patient was first observed to feel nauseated on 12th August 1993. In the same way, a "?" should be placed in front of the end date when entering the last day of observation.

If you have data on a patient going back to a time before the accident they will, of cause, be helpful. This is especially true in the case of numeric data, e. g., concentration of granulocytes. Please enter the available data in the manner as requested by the respective forms.

Miscellaneous

Topology

The location coding with an exemplary anatomical figure is found in chapter 6.

Lists

If there is a box where you can enter more then one item, e. g. for the location coding (example see below), please be sure to separate the items by using a comma "," followed by one space.

2.3.4 External Contamination

yes ☒, no ☐, unknown ☐, if yes please fill in the subsequent table

Part of the Body	Date and Time	Dose Rate [mSv/h]
1, 2L, 3L, 4L1	12.08.1993 13:00	5

Fig. 12   Coded Localisation given as a list in one box

6.5 Skin Burns

Date and Time	Localisation (see 6.2)	Degree (see 6.1)	Surface [% body surf.]	Surface [cm²]
28.04.1986	1F, 3L, 3R	0.5	5	

Fig. 13   Coded Localisation given as a list in one box

This applies to skin burns also. For the sake of convenience you may choose to list all localisations, for which the same degree is relevant, in one line.

Finally, the authors wish to thank you very much for your co-operation.

On behalf of the authors

Dirk Densow, M. D.

Main Part of the Questionnaire

TABLE OF CONTENTS

1. General Data on the Irradiated Patient

1.1 Demographic Data

family name (optional)							
given name (optional)							
code (of acc.)*							
ID-no**							
DB-ID-no	(to be added by the documentary)						
sex		male ☐			female ☐		
ethnicity	caucasian ☐		oriental ☐	negro ☐		other ☐	
if other please specify							
age at the time of the accident [yy]			date of birth [dd.mm.yyyy]				
length of the body [cm]							
home address							
telephone			telefax				

*　code - name of the accident in terms of the person who has first described the accident or code name as used for publication, e. g., code Y-12 -for the accident at Oak Ridge, Y-12 plant, 1958, code Chernobyl -for the accident at - Chernobyl Power Plant, 1986

**　ID-No. - identifying the patient for the respective hospital without revealing the patient's identity to the public., Patient A -for the accident at - Oak Ridge, Y-12 plant, 1958, UPN 1006 - for the accident at Chernobyl Power Plant, 1986

1.2 Occupation at the Time of the Accident

occupational activities at the time of the accident	
employer	
address	
telephone		telefax	

1.3   History at the Time of the Accident

Diagnosis	ICD-No.

The ICD-numbers should be given in case they are available for the respective diagnoses, if they are not available the fields should be left vacant.
If necessary please attach additional sheets here

1.4   Institutions Involved in Patient Care and Database Recording

1.4.1   Primary Care Institution Keeping the Patient's Medical Records

name			
address			
telephone		telefax	

1.4.2   Definitive Care Institution

name			
address			
telephone		telefax	

1.4.3   Physician Submitting the Case to the Registry

name			
address			
telephone		telefax	

1.4.4   Source of Compilation

the submission was completed from original case report of 1.4.2 or 1.4.3	☐	the submission was completed from literature (see also: "8.5 References")	☐
the submission was completed from other sources			☐
if yes, please specify here			
date of compilation [dd.mm.yyyy]		Please check consistency with Chptr. 5	

2.   Accident Information and Personal Exposure Conditions

2.1   Accident Description

For the Conversion to SI Units please refer to annex 8.2, for the orders of magnitude refer to annex 8.3.

2.1.1   Country

2.1.2   City

2.1.3   Location (Factory etc.) of the Accident

name	
address	
telephone		telefax	

2.1.4   Begin and End of the Accident

begin date and time [dd.mm.yyyy] [hh:mm]		end date and time [dd.mm.yyyy] [hh:mm]	

2.1.5   Proprietor of the Radiation Source

name	
address	
telephone		telefax	

2.1.6   General Description of the Accident

If more space is required, please attach more sheets here!

2.1.7 Number of Persons Involved

with clinical consequences		without clinical consequences, (WBI dose ≥ 0.25 Sv estimated)		without clinical consequences, (WBI dose 0.05 - 0.25 Sv estimated)	

2.1.8 IAEA Nuclear Event Scale

level, see annex 8.1		if necessary, please specify	

2.2 SOURCE OF IRRADIATION

2.2.1 Critical Chain Reaction   ☐ if yes please continue

critical assembly	☐	reactor	☐
liquid material	☐	dose rate on 1 m distance from centre of critical zone [Gy/h]	

2.2.2 Reactor Accident with Consecutive Emission   ☐ if yes please continue

dose rate, if given [Gy/h]		date and time of measurement [dd.mm.yyyy] [hh:mm]	
specify method of measurement			
specify place of measurement			

2.2.3 Nuclear Explosion   ☐ if yes please continue

in the air	☐	trace of fall-out	☐
dose rate, if given [Gy/h]			
specify method of measurement			
specify place of measurement			

2.2.4 Sealed Source   ☐ if yes please continue

radionuclide(s)*		activity [Bq]	
dose rate (at dist. of 1 m) [Gy/h]		length [cm]	
width [cm]		height [cm]	

*) e.g., ^{60}Co, ^{92}Ir etc.

2.2.5   Unsealed Source   ☐ if yes please continue

radionuclide(s)		activity [Bq]	
please specify mode of release			
please specify pattern of release			

2.2.6   X-ray Equipment   ☐ if yes please continue

current [mA]		voltage [kV]	
filter(s)			
other, please specify			

2.2.7   Accelerators   ☐ if yes please continue

kind of accelerator			
kind of particles		energy [MeV]	
width of the radiation field [cm]		height of the radiation field [cm]	
other, please specify			

2.2.8   Other Sources than 2.2.1 - 2.2.7   ☐ if yes please continue

other, please specify	

2.3   PERSONAL EXPOSURE CONDITIONS

2.3.1   Begin and End of Exposure

begin date and time [dd.mm.yyyy] [hh:mm]		end date and time [dd.mm.yyyy] [hh:mm]	
fractionated	yes ☐ no ☐ unknown ☐	if yes, please specify	

2.3.2   Individual Description of the Accident

If more space is required, please attach more sheets here!

2.3.3 External Irradiation

yes ☐, no ☐, unknown ☐, if yes please fill in the subsequent table

☞ Please use for coding of body surface the numbers of chapters 6.2 to 6.4, and give a scheme (see 3., below) of the location of the source and the person with respect to time and fill in the subsequent table

1. radiation geometry and data on shielding

Distance from Source [m]	Duration of Exposure [h:m:s]	Movement Relative to Source F OS DS[†]	Radiation Shield Yes, No, Uk	Type of Radiation Shield	Protected Part of the Body[‡]
> 2		☐ ☐ ☐	☐ ☐ ☐		
1 - 2		☐ ☐ ☐	☐ ☐ ☐		
0,5 - 1		☐ ☐ ☐	☐ ☐ ☐		
0.1 - 0.5		☐ ☐ ☐	☐ ☐ ☐		
< 0.1 *		☐ ☐ ☐	☐ ☐ ☐		

*) on body surface or in clothes (e.g. pocket etc.)
†) F - without moving (e.g., "flash")
OS - unilateral movement or standstill
DS - exposure from different sides
‡) For coding please use numbers of chapter 6.2 to 6.4

2. pattern of dose distribution as an overall judgement (check one box please)
2.1 homogeneous exposure ....☐
2.2 homogeneous exposure of bone marrow with local over-exposure (e. g. skin or extremities) ....☐
2.3 inhomogeneous exposure of bone marrow with local over-exposure (e. g. skin or extremities) ....☐
2.4 partial body exposure ....☐
2.5 local over-exposure (e. g. skin or extremities)..☐

3. scheme (if necessary)

If more space is required, please attach more sheets here!

2.3.4   External Contamination

yes ☐, no ☐, unknown ☐, if yes please fill in the subsequent table

Part of the Body [‡]	Date and Time	Dose Rate [mSv/h]
.		

[‡])   For coding please use numbers of chapter 6.2 to 6.4

2.3.5   Internal Contamination

yes ☐, no ☐, unknown ☐, if yes please fill in the subsequent table

way of intake	
radionuclide(s) and distribution	
solubility of radio-active compound(s)	

2.3.6   Evaluation of the Average Total Body Dose

yes ☐, no ☐, unknown ☐, if yes please fill in the subsequent table

Type of Measurement	Date and Time of Sampling or Begin of Evaluation	Date and Time of Receiving Results	Dose [Sv]
average total body dose			
direct measurement			
calculation			
chromosomal aberration analysis in peripheral blood lymphocytes			
chromosomal aberration analysis in bone marrow cells			
blood cell counts			
lymphocytes			
granulocytes			
paramagnetic resonance (PMR)			
teeth enamel			
other samples			
other methods			

2.3.7   Evaluation of Local Doses

yes ☐, no ☐, unknown ☐, if yes please fill in the subsequent table

Part of the Body ‡	Date and Time of Sampling or Begin of Evaluation	Date and Time of Receiving Results	Dose [Sv]	Method*

‡)   For coding please use numbers of chapter 6.2 to 6.4
*)   a - dosimetry, b - calculation, c - PMR, d - biological dosimetry (e.g., chromosomal aberration analysis)

2.3.8   Evaluation of Doses of Internal Exposure

yes ☐, no ☐, unknown ☐, if yes please fill in the subsequent table

Site*	Whole Body Counting	Organ Measure- ment	Excretion Measure- ment	Date and Time	Activity [Bq]	Dose [Sv]
	☐	☐	☐			
	☐	☐	☐			
	☐	☐	☐			
	☐	☐	☐			
	☐	☐	☐			
	☐	☐	☐			
	☐	☐	☐			
	☐	☐	☐			
	☐	☐	☐			
	☐	☐	☐			
	☐	☐	☐			
	☐	☐	☐			

*) please indicate which part or organ has been evaluated (e. g., total-body, head, thyroid etc.)

3   Clinical Data After Exposure

☞   Before filling in the questionnaire please read the Introduction carefully!

3.1   Primary Reaction

3.1.1   Dyspeptic Symptoms and Enlargement of Parotid Glands

all no ☐, all unknown ☐

Symptom	yes	no	uk	Begin (Date & Time)	End (Date & Time)	Maximum (Date & Time)	Degree
nausea	☐	☐	☐				
vomiting	☐	☐	☐				
abdominal pain	☐	☐	☐				
diarrhoea	☐	☐	☐				
enlargement of parotid glands	☐	☐	☐				
	☐	☐	☐				

3.1.2 Primary Skin Erythema and Hyperaemia of Mucous Membranes

all no ☐, all unknown ☐

Location	yes	no	uk	Begin (Date & Time)	End (Date & Time)	Maximum (Date & Time)	Degree
head and neck	☐	☐	☐				
upper part of body	☐	☐	☐				
arms	☐	☐	☐				
hands	☐	☐	☐				
lower part of body	☐	☐	☐				
legs	☐	☐	☐				
feet	☐	☐	☐				
oropharyngeal	☐	☐	☐				
	☐	☐	☐				

3.1.3 General Neurocirculatory Symptoms and Signs

all no ☐, all unknown ☐

Symptom/Sign	yes	no	uk	Begin (Date & Time)	End (Date & Time)	Maximum (Date & Time)	Degree
tachycardia (>100/min)	☐	☐	☐				
hypertension (>160/90)	☐	☐	☐				
hypotension (<100/60)	☐	☐	☐				
elevated BT (>38° C)	☐	☐	☐				
fatigue	☐	☐	☐				
headache	☐	☐	☐				
	☐	☐	☐				

3.2 Involvement of the Nervous System and the Eyes

3.2.1 Diagnostic Procedures for Central and Peripheral Nervous System

all no ☐, all unknown ☐

1. EEG .... yes ☐, no ☐, unknown ☐, if yes please add xerocopy
2. CT .... yes ☐, no ☐, unknown ☐, if yes please add xerocopy
3. NMR... yes ☐, no ☐, unknown ☐, if yes please add xerocopy
4. sonogram .... yes ☐, no ☐, unknown ☐, if yes please add xerocopy
5. visually evoked potentials... yes ☐, no ☐, unknown ☐, if yes please add xerocopy
6. EMG and ENG.. yes ☐, no ☐, unknown ☐, if yes please add xerocopy
7. biopsy.. yes ☐, no ☐, unknown ☐, if yes please add xerocopy
8. others .... yes ☐, no ☐, unknown ☐, if yes please add xerocopy,

if yes, please specify..

3.2.2 Impairment of Central and Peripheral Nervous System

1. symptoms and signs related to the brain, all no ☐, all unknown ☐

Symptom/Sign	yes	no	uk	Begin (Date & Time)	End (Date & Time)	Maximum (Date & Time)	Degree
diffuse headache	☐	☐	☐				
arching headache	☐	☐	☐				
dizziness	☐	☐	☐				
Kernig's sign	☐	☐	☐				
Brudzinski's sign	☐	☐	☐				
dolorous pressure sensitivity of neural points of the skull	☐	☐	☐				
temporal disorientation	☐	☐	☐				
somnolent state	☐	☐	☐				
coma	☐	☐	☐				
papillary stasis	☐	☐	☐				
papillary oedema	☐	☐	☐				
	☐	☐	☐				
	☐	☐	☐				

2. disturbances of reflexes (1), all no ☐, all unknown ☐

Symptom/Sign	yes	no	uk	Begin (Date & Time)	End (Date & Time)	Maximum (Date & Time)	Degree
hyporeflex. conjunctival reflex (L)	☐	☐	☐				
hyporeflex. conjunctival reflex (R)	☐	☐	☐				
hyporeflex. corneal reflex (L)	☐	☐	☐				
hyporeflex. corneal reflex (R)	☐	☐	☐				
hyporeflex. carpo-radial reflex (L)	☐	☐	☐				
hyporeflex. carpo-radial reflex (R)	☐	☐	☐				
hyperreflex. carpo-radial reflex (L)	☐	☐	☐				
hyperreflex. carpo-radial reflex (R)	☐	☐	☐				
hyporeflex. triceps tendon reflex (L)	☐	☐	☐				
hyporeflex. triceps tendon reflex (R)	☐	☐	☐				
hyperreflex. triceps tendon reflex (L)	☐	☐	☐				

2. disturbances of reflexes (2), all no ☐ , all unknown ☐

Symptom/Sign	yes	no	uk	Begin (Date & Time)	End (Date & Time)	Maximum (Date & Time)	Degree
hyperreflex. triceps tendon reflex (R)	☐	☐	☐				
hyporeflex. abdominal reflex (L)	☐	☐	☐				
hyporeflex. abdominal reflex (R)	☐	☐	☐				
hyporeflex. cremaster reflex (L)	☐	☐	☐				
hyporeflex. cremaster reflex (R)	☐	☐	☐				
hyporeflex. patellar reflex (L)	☐	☐	☐				
hyporeflex. patellar reflex (R)	☐	☐	☐				
hyperreflex. patellar reflex (L)	☐	☐	☐				
hyperreflex. patellar reflex (R)	☐	☐	☐				
hyporeflex. Achilles tendon reflex (L)	☐	☐	☐				
hyporeflex. Achilles tendon reflex (R)	☐	☐	☐				
hyperreflex. Achilles tendon reflex (L)	☐	☐	☐				
hyperreflex. Achilles tendon reflex (R)	☐	☐	☐				
pathologic foot reflexes (L)	☐	☐	☐				
pathologic foot reflexes (R)	☐	☐	☐				
	☐	☐	☐				
	☐	☐	☐				

3. disturbances of motor functions (1), all no ☐ , all unknown ☐

Symptom/Sign	yes	no	uk	Begin (Date & Time)	End (Date & Time)	Maximum (Date & Time)	Degree
hypotens. muscles of upper extremities (L)	☐	☐	☐				
hypotens. muscles of upper extremities (R)	☐	☐	☐				
hypotens. muscles of lower extremities (L)	☐	☐	☐				
hypotens. muscles of lower extremities (R)	☐	☐	☐				
hypertens. muscles of upper extremities (L)	☐	☐	☐				
hypertens. muscles of upper extremities (R)	☐	☐	☐				
hypertens. muscles of lower extremities (L)	☐	☐	☐				

3. disturbances of motor functions (2), all no ☐, all unknown ☐

Symptom/Sign	yes	no	uk	Begin (Date & Time)	End (Date & Time)	Maximum (Date & Time)	Degree
hypertens. muscles of lower extremities (R)	☐	☐	☐				
tonic cramps (L)	☐	☐	☐				
tonic cramps (R)	☐	☐	☐				
clonic cramps (L)	☐	☐	☐				
clonic cramps (R)	☐	☐	☐				
static ataxia (L)	☐	☐	☐				
static ataxia (R)	☐	☐	☐				
spastic muscular contraction (L)	☐	☐	☐				
spastic muscular contraction (R)	☐	☐	☐				
disturbed finger-nose test (L)	☐	☐	☐				
disturbed finger-nose test (R)	☐	☐	☐				
disturbed knee-heel test (L)	☐	☐	☐				
disturbed knee-heel test (R)	☐	☐	☐				
incomplete paralysis of upp. extremities (L)	☐	☐	☐				
incomplete paralysis of upp. extremities (R)	☐	☐	☐				
incomplete paralysis of low. extremities (L)	☐	☐	☐				
incomplete paralysis of low. extremities (R)	☐	☐	☐				
paralysis of upper extremities (L)	☐	☐	☐				
paralysis of upper extremities (R)	☐	☐	☐				
paralysis of lower extremities (L)	☐	☐	☐				
paralysis of lower extremities (R)	☐	☐	☐				

4. disturbances of sensation (1), all no ☐, all unknown ☐

Symptom/Sign	yes	no	uk	Begin (Date & Time)	End (Date & Time)	Maximum (Date & Time)	Degree
hypoaesthesia of head and neck (L)	☐	☐	☐				
hypoaesthesia of head and neck (R)	☐	☐	☐				
hyperaesthesia of head and neck (L)	☐	☐	☐				
hyperaesthesia of head and neck (R)	☐	☐	☐				
hypoaesthesia of upper extremities (L)	☐	☐	☐				

4. disturbances of sensation (2), all no ☐, all unknown ☐

Symptom/Sign	yes	no	uk	Begin (Date & Time)	End (Date & Time)	Maximum (Date & Time)	Degree
hypoaesthesia of upper extremities (R)	☐	☐	☐				
hyperaesthesia of upper extremities (L)	☐	☐	☐				
hyperaesthesia of upper extremities (R)	☐	☐	☐				
hypoaesthesia of trunk (L)	☐	☐	☐				
hypoaesthesia of trunk (R)	☐	☐	☐				
hyperaesthesia of trunk (L)	☐	☐	☐				
hyperaesthesia of trunk (R)	☐	☐	☐				
hypoaesthesia of lower extremities (L)	☐	☐	☐				
hypoaesthesia of lower extremities (R)	☐	☐	☐				
hyperaesthesia of lower extremities (L)	☐	☐	☐				
hyperaesthesia of lower extremities (R)	☐	☐	☐				
disturb. propriocept. sens. upp. extrem. (L)	☐	☐	☐				
disturb. propriocept. sens. upp. extrem. (R)	☐	☐	☐				
disturb. propriocept. sens. low. extrem. (L)	☐	☐	☐				
disturb. propriocept. sens. low. extrem. (R)	☐	☐	☐				
	☐	☐	☐				
	☐	☐	☐				

5. disturbances of autonomous nervous system, all no ☐, all unknown ☐

Symptom/Sign	yes	no	uk	Begin (Date & Time)	End (Date & Time)	Maximum (Date & Time)	Degree
reduced pulse rate after turning head (≥ 10)	☐	☐	☐				
reduced pulse rate after orthostasis (≥ 10)	☐	☐	☐				
incr. pulse rate after minimal work (≥ 20)	☐	☐	☐				
attacks of sweating	☐	☐	☐				
dizzy spell	☐	☐	☐				
	☐	☐	☐				

3.2.3   Lesions of Eyes

1.   lesions of eyelids and eyebrows, all no ☐, all unknown ☐

Symptom/Sign	yes	no	uk	Begin (Date & Time)	End (Date & Time)	Maximum (Date & Time)	Degree
primary erythema (L)	☐	☐	☐				
primary erythema (R)	☐	☐	☐				
second. erythema and pigment. (L)	☐	☐	☐				
second. erythema and pigment. (R)	☐	☐	☐				
radiation erosions and ulcers (L)	☐	☐	☐				
radiation erosions and ulcers (R)	☐	☐	☐				
epilation of eye lashes (L)	☐	☐	☐				
epilation of eye lashes (R)	☐	☐	☐				
epilation of eyebrows (L)	☐	☐	☐				
epilation of eyebrows (R)	☐	☐	☐				
	☐	☐	☐				
	☐	☐	☐				

2.   lesions of conjunctiva, all no ☐, all unknown ☐

Symptom/Sign	yes	no	uk	Begin (Date & Time)	End (Date & Time)	Maximum (Date & Time)	Degree
initial conjunctival hyperaemia (L)	☐	☐	☐				
initial conjunctival hyperaemia (R)	☐	☐	☐				
secondary hyperaemia (L)	☐	☐	☐				
secondary hyperaemia (R)	☐	☐	☐				
radiation erosions and ulcers (L)	☐	☐	☐				
radiation erosions and ulcers (R)	☐	☐	☐				
radiation conjunc-tivitis (L)	☐	☐	☐				
radiation conjunc-tivitis (R)	☐	☐	☐				
	☐	☐	☐				
	☐	☐	☐				

3. lesions of cornea and front eye chamber, all no ☐, all unknown ☐

Symptom/Sign	yes	no	uk	Begin (Date & Time)	End (Date & Time)	Maximum (Date & Time)	Degree
reduced cornea sensitivity (L)	☐	☐	☐				
reduced cornea sensitivity (R)	☐	☐	☐				
erosive keratitis (L)	☐	☐	☐				
erosive keratitis (R)	☐	☐	☐				
ulcer. keratitis (L)	☐	☐	☐				
ulcer. keratitis (R)	☐	☐	☐				
iritis (L)	☐	☐	☐				
iritis (R)	☐	☐	☐				
	☐	☐	☐				

4. lesions of lens, all no ☐, all unknown ☐

Symptom/Sign	yes	no	uk	Begin (Date & Time)	End (Date & Time)	Maximum (Date & Time)	Degree
cataract (L)	☐	☐	☐				
cataract (R)	☐	☐	☐				
	☐	☐	☐				

5. changes of eye fundus, all no ☐, all unknown ☐

Symptom/Sign	yes	no	uk	Begin (Date & Time)	End (Date & Time)	Maximum (Date & Time)	Degree
ext. of fundus blood vessel (L)	☐	☐	☐				
ext. of fundus blood vessel (R)	☐	☐	☐				
reduced pressure in A. centr. ret. (L)	☐	☐	☐				
reduced pressure in A. centr. ret. (R)	☐	☐	☐				
oedema of retina (L)	☐	☐	☐				
oedema of retina (R)	☐	☐	☐				
ret. haemorrhage (L)	☐	☐	☐				
ret. haemorrhage (R)	☐	☐	☐				
	☐	☐	☐				

3.3   Radiation Induced Lesions of Skin, its Appendices, and Underlying Tissues

3.3.1   Diagnostic Procedures

all no ☐, all unknown ☐

1. thermography .... yes ☐, no ☐, unknown ☐, if yes please add xerocopy
2. sonogram .... yes ☐, no ☐, unknown ☐, if yes please add xerocopy
3. NMR .... yes ☐, no ☐, unknown ☐, if yes please add xerocopy
4. CT .... yes ☐, no ☐, unknown ☐, if yes please add xerocopy
5. biopsy .... yes ☐, no ☐, unknown ☐, if yes please add xerocopy
6. others .... yes ☐, no ☐, unknown ☐, if yes please add xerocopy,

if yes, please specify ....

3.3.2   Radiation Induced Skin Lesions

yes ☐, no ☐, unknown ☐, if yes please continue

> ☞   Please insert detailed data on skin lesions, i. e., thermal burns and radiation lesions in chapter 6.5. Give a rough estimate at the time of the maximum of the lesions.

1. estimate of percentage of body surface with different degrees (for grading see following scheme) of skin burns

erythema	1	erythema and blisters	2
erosion	3	necrosis	4

Degree	Percentage	Sites ‡
1		
2		
3		
4		

‡)   For coding please use numbers of chapter 6.2 to 6.4

2. symptoms at the site of the most severe burns, all no ☐, all unknown ☐

Symptom/Sign	yes	no	uk	Begin (Date & Time)	End (Date & Time)	Maximum (Date & Time)	Degree
severe pain	☐	☐	☐				
marked oedema of underlying tissues	☐	☐	☐				
necrosis of underlying tissues	☐	☐	☐				
	☐	☐	☐				

3.3.3   Disturbances of Nails

all no ☐, all unknown ☐

Symptom/Sign	yes	no	uk	Begin (Date & Time)	End (Date & Time)	Maximum (Date & Time)	Degree
growth retardation	☐	☐	☐				
pigmentation	☐	☐	☐				
	☐	☐	☐				

3.3.4   Epilation

yes ☐, no ☐, unknown ☐, if yes please fill in the subsequent table

Site	Begin (Date & Time)	Epilation com, inc, uk+	Reversibility of Epilation yes, no, uk	If yes, Begin of Hair Growth (Date & Time)
head (L)		☐ ☐ ☐	☐ ☐ ☐	
head (R)		☐ ☐ ☐	☐ ☐ ☐	
beard (L)		☐ ☐ ☐	☐ ☐ ☐	
beard (R)		☐ ☐ ☐	☐ ☐ ☐	
axilla (L)		☐ ☐ ☐	☐ ☐ ☐	
axilla (R)		☐ ☐ ☐	☐ ☐ ☐	
chest (L)		☐ ☐ ☐	☐ ☐ ☐	
chest (R)		☐ ☐ ☐	☐ ☐ ☐	
pubis (L)		☐ ☐ ☐	☐ ☐ ☐	
pubis (R)		☐ ☐ ☐	☐ ☐ ☐	
legs (L)		☐ ☐ ☐	☐ ☐ ☐	
legs (R)		☐ ☐ ☐	☐ ☐ ☐	
		☐ ☐ ☐	☐ ☐ ☐	
		☐ ☐ ☐	☐ ☐ ☐	

+) com = complete; inc = incomplete; uk = unknown

3.3.5   **Amputation of Extremities**

yes ☐, no ☐, unknown ☐, if yes please fill in the subsequent table

Date and Time	Site ‡	Specification *

‡) For coding please use numbers of chapter 6.2 to 6.4
*) enter as free text

3.3.6   **Debridement of Necrotic Tissue**

yes ☐, no ☐, unknown ☐, if yes please fill in the subsequent table

Date and Time	Site ‡	Specification *

‡) For coding please use numbers of chapter 6.2 to 6.4
*) enter as free text

3.3.7   **Reconstructive Surgery due to Dermal Radiation Lesions**

yes ☐, no ☐, unknown ☐, if yes please fill in the subsequent table

Date and Time	Site ‡	Specification *

‡) For coding please use numbers of chapter 6.2 to 6.4
*) enter as free text

3.4   Bone Marrow Syndrome and Blood

☞   The normal values of the laboratory data should be given in annex 8.6.

☞   To insert data in the following tables please use one line for one sample only, even if the previous line has not been filled in completely. If you need more space we kindly request that you xerocopy the scheme for continuation (see annex 8.7). The numbers in the beginning of each row will help you to identify the corresponding rows on the right side of the table. They do not indicate numbers of days after exposure.
          If available please include patient's recent haematological data (before the exposure) in the beginning of the tables. Please use the appropriate format.

3.4.1   Peripheral Blood Count

yes ☐, no ☐, unknown ☐, if yes please continue

Peripheral Blood Count (1, left)

	Date and Time	RBC [Tera/l]	Haemo-globin [g/l]	Haema-tocrit [%]	MCV [femto-l]	Reticulo-cytes [%]	Platelets [Giga/l]	ESR [mm/h]	WBC [Giga/l]
1									
2									
3									
4									
5									
6									
7									
8									
9									
10									
11									
12									
13									
14									
15									
16									
17									
18									
19									
20									
21									
22									
23									
24									
25									
26									
27									
28									
29									
30									

Peripheral Blood Count (1, right)

	Granulo-cytes [Giga/l]	Lympho-cytes [Giga/l]									
1											
2											
3											
4											
5											
6											
7											
8											
9											
10											
11											
12											
13											
14											
15											
16											
17											
18											
19											
20											
21											
22											
23											
24											
25											
26											
27											
28											
29											
30											

Peripheral Blood Count (2, left)

	Date and Time	RBC [Tera/l]	Haemo-globin [g/l]	Haema-tocrit [%]	MCV [femto-l]	Reticulo-cytes [%]	Platelets [Giga/l]	ESR [mm/h]	WBC [Giga/l]
31									
32									
33									
34									
35									
36									
37									
38									
39									
40									
41									
42									
43									
44									
45									
46									
47									
48									
49									
50									
51									
52									
53									
54									
55									
56									
57									
58									
59									
60									

Peripheral Blood Count (2, right)

	Granulo-cytes [Giga/l]	Lympho-cytes [Giga/l]								
31										
32										
33										
34										
35										
36										
37										
38										
39										
40										
41										
42										
43										
44										
45										
46										
47										
48										
49										
50										
51										
52										
53										
54										
55										
56										
57										
58										
59										
60										

Peripheral Blood Count (3, left)

	Date and Time	RBC [Tera/l]	Haemo-globin [g/l]	Haema-tocrit [%]	MCV [femto-l]	Reticulo-cytes [%]	Platelets [Giga/l]	ESR [mm/h]	WBC [Giga/l]
61									
62									
63									
64									
65									
66									
67									
68									
69									
70									
71									
72									
73									
74									
75									
76									
77									
78									
79									
80									
81									
82									
83									
84									
85									
86									
87									
88									
89									
90									

Peripheral Blood Count (3, right)

	Granulo-cytes [Giga/l]	Lympho-cytes [Giga/l]									
61											
62											
63											
64											
65											
66											
67											
68											
69											
70											
71											
72											
73											
74											
75											
76											
77											
78											
79											
80											
81											
82											
83											
84											
85											
86											
87											
88											
89											
90											

3.4.2   **Peripheral Blood Smear**   yes ☐, no ☐, unknown ☐, if yes please continue

Peripheral Blood Smear (1 left)

	Date and Time	Blasts	Myelo-blasts	Promye-locytes	Myelo-cyte	Metamy-elocyte	Band Neutr. Granulo-cyte	Segm. Neutr. Granulo-cyte	Lympho-cyte
1									
2									
3									
4									
5									
6									
7									
8									
9									
10									
11									
12									
13									
14									
15									
16									
17									
18									
19									
20									
21									
22									
23									
24									
25									
26									
27									
28									
29									
30									

Peripheral Blood Smear (1 right)

	Mono-cyte	Eosino-phils	Baso-phils	Plasma-cells	Mitotic Conn. A-nom. of RBC	Mitotic Conn. Anom. of Granul.	Mitotic Conn. Anom. of Lympho.	Gigantic Granulo-cytes	Atypical/ Unidenti-fied		
1											
2											
3											
4											
5											
6											
7											
8											
9											
10											
11											
12											
13											
14											
15											
16											
17											
18											
19											
20											
21											
22											
23											
24											
25											
26											
27											
28											
29											
30											

Peripheral Blood Smear (2 left)

	Date and Time	Blasts	Myelo-blasts	Promye-locytes	Myelo-cyte	Metamy-elocyte	Band Neutr. Granulo-cyte	Segm. Neutr. Granulo-cyte	Lympho-cyte
31									
32									
33									
34									
35									
36									
37									
38									
39									
40									
41									
42									
43									
44									
45									
46									
47									
48									
49									
50									
51									
52									
53									
54									
55									
56									
57									
58									
59									
60									

Peripheral Blood Smear (2 right)

	Mono-cyte	Eosino-phils	Baso-phils	Plasma-cells	Mitotic Conn. A-nom. of RBC	Mitotic Conn. Anom. of Granul.	Mitotic Conn. Anom. of Lympho.	Gigantic Granulo-cytes	Atypical/ Unidenti-fied		
31											
32											
33											
34											
35											
36											
37											
38											
39											
40											
41											
42											
43											
44											
45											
46											
47											
48											
49											
50											
51											
52											
53											
54											
55											
56											
57											
58											
59											
60											

Peripheral Blood Smear (3 left)

	Date and Time	Blasts	Myelo-blasts	Promye-locytes	Myelo-cyte	Metamy-elocyte	Band Neutr. Granulo-cyte	Segm. Neutr. Granulo-cyte	Lympho-cyte
61									
62									
63									
64									
65									
66									
67									
68									
69									
70									
71									
72									
73									
74									
75									
76									
77									
78									
79									
80									
81									
82									
83									
84									
85									
86									
87									
88									
89									
90									

Peripheral Blood Smear (3 right)

	Mono-cyte	Eosino-phils	Baso-phils	Plasma-cells	Mitotic Conn. A-nom. of RBC	Mitotic Conn. Anom. of Granul.	Mitotic Conn. Anom. of Lympho.	Gigantic Granulo-cytes	Atypical/ Unidenti-fied		
61											
62											
63											
64											
65											
66											
67											
68											
69											
70											
71											
72											
73											
74											
75											
76											
77											
78											
79											
80											
81											
82											
83											
84											
85											
86											
87											
88											
89											
90											

3.4.3 **Bone Marrow Examination**   yes ☐, no ☐, unknown ☐, if yes please continue

Date and Time					
Punctuation Site*		VC __			
Myelopoietic Tissue					
Number of Nucleated Cells					
Mit. Conn. Anom. of Erythropoiesis					
Mit. Conn. Anom. of Myeolopoiesis					
Blast					
Myeloblast					
Promyelocyte					
Myelocyte					
Metamyelocyte					
Band Neutrophil Granulocyte					
Segm. Neutrophil Granulocyte					
Basophil					
Eosinophilic Myelocyte					
Eosinophilic Metamyelocyte					
Eosinophil					
Lymphocyte					
Monocyte					
Plasmacell					
Makrophages					
Normoblast Mitoses					
Erythroblast					
Basophilic Normoblast					
Polynormoblast					
Oxyphilic Normoblast					
Megakaryocytes					
Gigantic Neutrophils					
Degenerated Neutrophils					
Degenerated Normoblasts					
Jolly's Bodies					

*)punctuation site for bone marrow cells

Sternum	ST	Spina iliaca ant. sup. sin.	AS	Spina iliaca ant. sup. dex.	AD
Spina iliaca post. sup. sin.	PS	Spina iliaca post. sup. dex.	PD		
Proc. spinosus vert. cerv. no. ...	VC __	Proc. spinosus vert. thor. no. ..	VT __	Proc. spinosus vert. lumb. no. ..	VL __

3.4.4 Cytogenetic Data

yes ☐, no ☐, unknown ☐, if yes please continue

Date and Time					
Material*	VC __		VT __		VL __
Number of Cells Scored					
No. of Cells with Chromosomal Aberr.					
No. of C. with Chromatide Aberrations					
No. of Aberrant Cells					
Dicentrics					
Rings					
Acentrics					
Chromatide Breaks					
Chrom. Exchanges					
Atypical Chromosomes					
Sex Chromosomes XX/XY					
No. of Cells with Aneupleoidy					
Aneupleoidy No. of Chromosomes					
No. of Cells with 0 Dicentric					
No. of Cells with 1 Dicentric					
No. of Cells with 2 Dicentrics					
No. of Cells with 3 Dicentrics					
No. of Cells with 4 Dicentrics					
No. of Cells with 5 Dicentrics					
No. of Cells with 6 Dicentrics					
No. of Cells with 7 Dicentrics					
No. of Cells with 8 Dicentrics					
No. of Cells with 9 Dicentrics					
No. of Cells with 10 Dicentrics					
No. of Cells with 11 Dicentrics					
No. of Cells with 12 Dicentrics					
No. of Cells with ≥ 13 Dicentrics					

*)material and punctuation site for bone marrow cells

PHA-stim. periph. blood lymphocytes	PBL	PHA-stim. bone marrow lympho.	PML	native bone marrow cells	BMC
punctuation sites		Sternum	ST	Spina iliaca ant. sup. sin.	AS
Spina iliaca ant. sup. dex.	AD	Spina iliaca post. sup. sin.	PS	Spina iliaca post. sup. dex.	PD
Proc. spinosus vert. cerv. no. ...	VC __	Proc. spinosus vert. thor. no. ..	VT __	Proc. spinosus vert. lumb. no. ..	VL __

3.4.5   **Biochemical Data**

Biochemical Data (1, left).

yes ☐, no ☐, unknown ☐, if yes please continue

Important notice: This table extends on 4 pages, this is page 1.

	Date and Time	Bilirubin, total [μmol/l]	Bilirubin, direct [μmol/l]	ALT [U/l]	AST [U/l]	γ-GT [U/l]	LDH (total) [U/l]	LDH-I [U/l]	LDH-II [U/l]
1									
2									
3									
4									
5									
6									
7									
8									
9									
10									
11									
12									
13									
14									
15									
16									
17									
18									
19									
20									
21									
22									
23									
24									
25									
26									
27									
28									
29									
30									

Biochemical Data (1, middle-left).

Important notice: This table extends on 4 pages, this is page 2.

	LDH-III [U/l]	LDH-IV [U/l]	LDH-V [U/l]	Ach.-esterase [U/l]	Alk. Pho-sphatase [U/l]	CK [U/l]	CK-MB [U/l]	Amylase Serum [U/l]	Chole-sterol [mmol/l]	Urea [mmol/l]	Uric Acid [µmol/l]
1											
2											
3											
4											
5											
6											
7											
8											
9											
10											
11											
12											
13											
14											
15											
16											
17											
18											
19											
20											
21											
22											
23											
24											
25											
26											
27											
28											
29											
30											

Biochemical Data (1, middle-right).

Important notice: This table extends on 4 pages, this is page 3.

	Date and Time	Glucose - Serum [mmol/l]	Creati- nine [μmol/l]	Total Protein [g/l]	Albumin [g/l]	α1- Globulin [g/l]	α2- Globulin [g/l]	β- Globulin [g/l]	γ- Globulin [g/l]
1									
2									
3									
4									
5									
6									
7									
8									
9									
10									
11									
12									
13									
14									
15									
16									
17									
18									
19									
20									
21									
22									
23									
24									
25									
26									
27									
28									
29									
30									

Biochemical Data (1, right).

Important notice: This table extends on 4 pages, this is page 4.

	K [mmol/l]	Na [mmol/l]	Ca [mmol/l]	Fe [μmol/l]	S-Phos-phorus [mmol/l]	Chloride [mmol/l]					
1											
2											
3											
4											
5											
6											
7											
8											
9											
10											
11											
12											
13											
14											
15											
16											
17											
18											
19											
20											
21											
22											
23											
24											
25											
26											
27											
28											
29											
30											

3.4.6   **Haemostatic Parameters**   yes ☐, no ☐, unknown ☐, if yes please continue

Haemostatic Parameters (1, left)

	Date and Time	PTT [s]	PT (QUICK) [%]	TT [s]	Fibri-nogen [μmol/l]	Ethanol-Test [#]	Protamin Sulphate Test [n#]	Retrac-tion-Test	Bleeding-Time DUKE [m]
1									
2									
3									
4									
5									
6									
7									
8									
9									
10									
11									
12									
13									
14									
15									
16									
17									
18									
19									
20									
21									
22									
23									
24									
25									
26									
27									
28									
29									
30									

Haemostatic Parameters (1, right)

	Factor II [%]	Factor V [%]	Factor VIII [%]	Factor IX [%]	Factor X [%]	Fibrinol. Activity [min]	Anti-thrombin III [U/l]				
1											
2											
3											
4											
5											
6											
7											
8											
9											
10											
11											
12											
13											
14											
15											
16											
17											
18											
19											
20											
21											
22											
23											
24											
25											
26											
27											
28											
29											
30											

3.4.7   Immunological and Immunohaematological Tests

yes ☐, no ☐, unknown ☐, if yes please continue

Immunological Parameters (1, left)

	Date and Time	C-React. Protein [g/l]	T-Cells [%]	T-Helper [%]	T-Sup-pressor [%]	B-Cells [%]	IgG [g/l]	IgA [g/l]	IgM [g/l]
1									
2									
3									
4									
5									
6									
7									
8									
9									
10									
11									
12									
13									
14									
15									
16									
17									
18									
19									
20									
21									
22									
23									
24									
25									
26									
27									
28									
29									
30									

Immunological Parameters (1, right)

	Comple-ment [g/l]									
1										
2										
3										
4										
5										
6										
7										
8										
9										
10										
11										
12										
13										
14										
15										
16										
17										
18										
19										
20										
21										
22										
23										
24										
25										
26										
27										
28										
29										
30										

Immunohaematological Tests(1, left)

	Date and Time	Coomb's direct pos , neg	Coomb's indirect pos , neg	Aggreg. Agglutin. Test pos, neg	Isohaem-aggluti-nin α [1:n]	Isohaem-aggluti-nin β [1:n]			
1		☐ ☐	☐ ☐	☐ ☐					
2		☐ ☐	☐ ☐	☐ ☐					
3		☐ ☐	☐ ☐	☐ ☐					
4		☐ ☐	☐ ☐	☐ ☐					
5		☐ ☐	☐ ☐	☐ ☐					
6		☐ ☐	☐ ☐	☐ ☐					
7		☐ ☐	☐ ☐	☐ ☐					
8		☐ ☐	☐ ☐	☐ ☐					
9		☐ ☐	☐ ☐	☐ ☐					
10		☐ ☐	☐ ☐	☐ ☐					
11		☐ ☐	☐ ☐	☐ ☐					
12		☐ ☐	☐ ☐	☐ ☐					
13		☐ ☐	☐ ☐	☐ ☐					
14		☐ ☐	☐ ☐	☐ ☐					
15		☐ ☐	☐ ☐	☐ ☐					
16		☐ ☐	☐ ☐	☐ ☐					
17		☐ ☐	☐ ☐	☐ ☐					
18		☐ ☐	☐ ☐	☐ ☐					
19		☐ ☐	☐ ☐	☐ ☐					
20		☐ ☐	☐ ☐	☐ ☐					
21		☐ ☐	☐ ☐	☐ ☐					
22		☐ ☐	☐ ☐	☐ ☐					
23		☐ ☐	☐ ☐	☐ ☐					
24		☐ ☐	☐ ☐	☐ ☐					
25		☐ ☐	☐ ☐	☐ ☐					
26		☐ ☐	☐ ☐	☐ ☐					
27		☐ ☐	☐ ☐	☐ ☐					
28		☐ ☐	☐ ☐	☐ ☐					
29		☐ ☐	☐ ☐	☐ ☐					
30		☐ ☐	☐ ☐	☐ ☐					

Immunohaematological Tests(1, right)

1											
2											
3											
4											
5											
6											
7											
8											
9											
10											
11											
12											
13											
14											
15											
16											
17											
18											
19											
20											
21											
22											
23											
24											
25											
26											
27											
28											
29											
30											

3.4.8 Microbiological Analysis

yes ☐, no ☐, unknown ☐, if yes please continue

Result of Cultures(1)

	Date and Time	Blood culture bac fung neg	Urine culture bac fung neg	Stool culture bac fung neg	Throat cult. bac fung neg		
1		☐ ☐ ☐	☐ ☐ ☐	☐ ☐ ☐	☐ ☐ ☐	☐ ☐ ☐	☐ ☐ ☐
2		☐ ☐ ☐	☐ ☐ ☐	☐ ☐ ☐	☐ ☐ ☐	☐ ☐ ☐	☐ ☐ ☐
3		☐ ☐ ☐	☐ ☐ ☐	☐ ☐ ☐	☐ ☐ ☐	☐ ☐ ☐	☐ ☐ ☐
4		☐ ☐ ☐	☐ ☐ ☐	☐ ☐ ☐	☐ ☐ ☐	☐ ☐ ☐	☐ ☐ ☐
5		☐ ☐ ☐	☐ ☐ ☐	☐ ☐ ☐	☐ ☐ ☐	☐ ☐ ☐	☐ ☐ ☐
6		☐ ☐ ☐	☐ ☐ ☐	☐ ☐ ☐	☐ ☐ ☐	☐ ☐ ☐	☐ ☐ ☐
7		☐ ☐ ☐	☐ ☐ ☐	☐ ☐ ☐	☐ ☐ ☐	☐ ☐ ☐	☐ ☐ ☐
8		☐ ☐ ☐	☐ ☐ ☐	☐ ☐ ☐	☐ ☐ ☐	☐ ☐ ☐	☐ ☐ ☐
9		☐ ☐ ☐	☐ ☐ ☐	☐ ☐ ☐	☐ ☐ ☐	☐ ☐ ☐	☐ ☐ ☐
10		☐ ☐ ☐	☐ ☐ ☐	☐ ☐ ☐	☐ ☐ ☐	☐ ☐ ☐	☐ ☐ ☐
11		☐ ☐ ☐	☐ ☐ ☐	☐ ☐ ☐	☐ ☐ ☐	☐ ☐ ☐	☐ ☐ ☐
12		☐ ☐ ☐	☐ ☐ ☐	☐ ☐ ☐	☐ ☐ ☐	☐ ☐ ☐	☐ ☐ ☐
13		☐ ☐ ☐	☐ ☐ ☐	☐ ☐ ☐	☐ ☐ ☐	☐ ☐ ☐	☐ ☐ ☐
14		☐ ☐ ☐	☐ ☐ ☐	☐ ☐ ☐	☐ ☐ ☐	☐ ☐ ☐	☐ ☐ ☐
15		☐ ☐ ☐	☐ ☐ ☐	☐ ☐ ☐	☐ ☐ ☐	☐ ☐ ☐	☐ ☐ ☐
16		☐ ☐ ☐	☐ ☐ ☐	☐ ☐ ☐	☐ ☐ ☐	☐ ☐ ☐	☐ ☐ ☐
17		☐ ☐ ☐	☐ ☐ ☐	☐ ☐ ☐	☐ ☐ ☐	☐ ☐ ☐	☐ ☐ ☐
18		☐ ☐ ☐	☐ ☐ ☐	☐ ☐ ☐	☐ ☐ ☐	☐ ☐ ☐	☐ ☐ ☐
19		☐ ☐ ☐	☐ ☐ ☐	☐ ☐ ☐	☐ ☐ ☐	☐ ☐ ☐	☐ ☐ ☐
20		☐ ☐ ☐	☐ ☐ ☐	☐ ☐ ☐	☐ ☐ ☐	☐ ☐ ☐	☐ ☐ ☐
21		☐ ☐ ☐	☐ ☐ ☐	☐ ☐ ☐	☐ ☐ ☐	☐ ☐ ☐	☐ ☐ ☐
22		☐ ☐ ☐	☐ ☐ ☐	☐ ☐ ☐	☐ ☐ ☐	☐ ☐ ☐	☐ ☐ ☐
23		☐ ☐ ☐	☐ ☐ ☐	☐ ☐ ☐	☐ ☐ ☐	☐ ☐ ☐	☐ ☐ ☐
24		☐ ☐ ☐	☐ ☐ ☐	☐ ☐ ☐	☐ ☐ ☐	☐ ☐ ☐	☐ ☐ ☐
25		☐ ☐ ☐	☐ ☐ ☐	☐ ☐ ☐	☐ ☐ ☐	☐ ☐ ☐	☐ ☐ ☐
26		☐ ☐ ☐	☐ ☐ ☐	☐ ☐ ☐	☐ ☐ ☐	☐ ☐ ☐	☐ ☐ ☐
27		☐ ☐ ☐	☐ ☐ ☐	☐ ☐ ☐	☐ ☐ ☐	☐ ☐ ☐	☐ ☐ ☐
28		☐ ☐ ☐	☐ ☐ ☐	☐ ☐ ☐	☐ ☐ ☐	☐ ☐ ☐	☐ ☐ ☐
29		☐ ☐ ☐	☐ ☐ ☐	☐ ☐ ☐	☐ ☐ ☐	☐ ☐ ☐	☐ ☐ ☐
30		☐ ☐ ☐	☐ ☐ ☐	☐ ☐ ☐	☐ ☐ ☐	☐ ☐ ☐	☐ ☐ ☐

Result of Cultures(2)

	Date and Time	Blood culture bac fung neg			Urine culture bac fung neg			Stool culture bac fung neg			Throat cult. bac fung neg								
31		☐	☐	☐	☐	☐	☐	☐	☐	☐	☐	☐	☐	☐	☐	☐	☐	☐	☐
32		☐	☐	☐	☐	☐	☐	☐	☐	☐	☐	☐	☐	☐	☐	☐	☐	☐	☐
33		☐	☐	☐	☐	☐	☐	☐	☐	☐	☐	☐	☐	☐	☐	☐	☐	☐	☐
34		☐	☐	☐	☐	☐	☐	☐	☐	☐	☐	☐	☐	☐	☐	☐	☐	☐	☐
35		☐	☐	☐	☐	☐	☐	☐	☐	☐	☐	☐	☐	☐	☐	☐	☐	☐	☐
36		☐	☐	☐	☐	☐	☐	☐	☐	☐	☐	☐	☐	☐	☐	☐	☐	☐	☐
37		☐	☐	☐	☐	☐	☐	☐	☐	☐	☐	☐	☐	☐	☐	☐	☐	☐	☐
38		☐	☐	☐	☐	☐	☐	☐	☐	☐	☐	☐	☐	☐	☐	☐	☐	☐	☐
39		☐	☐	☐	☐	☐	☐	☐	☐	☐	☐	☐	☐	☐	☐	☐	☐	☐	☐
40		☐	☐	☐	☐	☐	☐	☐	☐	☐	☐	☐	☐	☐	☐	☐	☐	☐	☐
41		☐	☐	☐	☐	☐	☐	☐	☐	☐	☐	☐	☐	☐	☐	☐	☐	☐	☐
42		☐	☐	☐	☐	☐	☐	☐	☐	☐	☐	☐	☐	☐	☐	☐	☐	☐	☐
43		☐	☐	☐	☐	☐	☐	☐	☐	☐	☐	☐	☐	☐	☐	☐	☐	☐	☐
44		☐	☐	☐	☐	☐	☐	☐	☐	☐	☐	☐	☐	☐	☐	☐	☐	☐	☐
45		☐	☐	☐	☐	☐	☐	☐	☐	☐	☐	☐	☐	☐	☐	☐	☐	☐	☐
46		☐	☐	☐	☐	☐	☐	☐	☐	☐	☐	☐	☐	☐	☐	☐	☐	☐	☐
47		☐	☐	☐	☐	☐	☐	☐	☐	☐	☐	☐	☐	☐	☐	☐	☐	☐	☐
48		☐	☐	☐	☐	☐	☐	☐	☐	☐	☐	☐	☐	☐	☐	☐	☐	☐	☐
49		☐	☐	☐	☐	☐	☐	☐	☐	☐	☐	☐	☐	☐	☐	☐	☐	☐	☐
50		☐	☐	☐	☐	☐	☐	☐	☐	☐	☐	☐	☐	☐	☐	☐	☐	☐	☐
51		☐	☐	☐	☐	☐	☐	☐	☐	☐	☐	☐	☐	☐	☐	☐	☐	☐	☐
52		☐	☐	☐	☐	☐	☐	☐	☐	☐	☐	☐	☐	☐	☐	☐	☐	☐	☐
53		☐	☐	☐	☐	☐	☐	☐	☐	☐	☐	☐	☐	☐	☐	☐	☐	☐	☐
54		☐	☐	☐	☐	☐	☐	☐	☐	☐	☐	☐	☐	☐	☐	☐	☐	☐	☐
55		☐	☐	☐	☐	☐	☐	☐	☐	☐	☐	☐	☐	☐	☐	☐	☐	☐	☐
56		☐	☐	☐	☐	☐	☐	☐	☐	☐	☐	☐	☐	☐	☐	☐	☐	☐	☐
57		☐	☐	☐	☐	☐	☐	☐	☐	☐	☐	☐	☐	☐	☐	☐	☐	☐	☐
58		☐	☐	☐	☐	☐	☐	☐	☐	☐	☐	☐	☐	☐	☐	☐	☐	☐	☐
59		☐	☐	☐	☐	☐	☐	☐	☐	☐	☐	☐	☐	☐	☐	☐	☐	☐	☐
60		☐	☐	☐	☐	☐	☐	☐	☐	☐	☐	☐	☐	☐	☐	☐	☐	☐	☐

Antibiogramm (1, left) †

Date and Time				
Source of Material				uk
Species				
No. of Microbes per g or ml of Material				
Drugs :				
1				
2				
3				
4				
5				
6				
7				
8				
9				
10				
11				
12				
13				
14				
15				
16				
17				
18				
19				
20				
21				
22				
23				
24				
25				
26				
27				
28				
29				
30				
31				

† **Please indicate the degree of sensitivity as follows:**

very sensitive   +   sensitive   o   not sensitive   -   unknown or not tested   uk

Antibiogramm (1, left) †

	very sensitive				
1					
2					
3					
4					
5					
6					
7					
8					
9					
10					
11					
12					
13					
14					
15					
16					
17					
18					
19					
20					
21					
22					
23					
24					
25					
26					
27					
28					
29					
30					
31					

† Please indicate the degree of sensitivity as follows:

| very sensitive | + | sensitive | o | not sensitive | - | unknown or not tested | uk |

3.4.9   Lesions of Bone Marrow

1. pancytopenia characteristic to radiation   yes ☐, no ☐, unknown ☐

2. clinical consequences thereof

2.1 haemorrhage   all no ☐, all unknown ☐, if so proceed to 2.2

☞   Please describe the severity of the haemorrhage by the scores as indicated in the manual.

Symptom/Sign	yes	no	uk	Begin (Date & Time)	End (Date & Time)	Maximum (Date & Time)	Degree
dermal haemorrhage	☐	☐	☐				
epistaxis	☐	☐	☐				
oral haemorrhage	☐	☐	☐				
conjunctival haemorrhage	☐	☐	☐				
retinal haemorrhage	☐	☐	☐				
cns haemorrhage	☐	☐	☐				
haematemesis	☐	☐	☐				
haemoptysis	☐	☐	☐				
melena	☐	☐	☐				
bloody diarrhoea	☐	☐	☐				
haematuria	☐	☐	☐				
metrorrhagia	☐	☐	☐				
wound haemorrhage	☐	☐	☐				
	☐	☐	☐				
	☐	☐	☐				
	☐	☐	☐				
	☐	☐	☐				
	☐	☐	☐				
	☐	☐	☐				
	☐	☐	☐				
	☐	☐	☐				
	☐	☐	☐				
	☐	☐	☐				

2.2   infection   yes ☐, no ☐, unknown ☐, if yes please continue

Diagnosis	B*	V	F	P	UK	Begin (Date & Time)	End (Date & Time)	Degree
septicaemia	☐	☐	☐	☐	☐			
pneumonia	☐	☐	☐	☐	☐			
necrotic enteropathy	☐	☐	☐	☐	☐			
oral infection	☐	☐	☐	☐	☐			
rhinitis	☐	☐	☐	☐	☐			
pharyngitis	☐	☐	☐	☐	☐			
tonsillitis	☐	☐	☐	☐	☐			
otitis	☐	☐	☐	☐	☐			
herpes simplex labialis		☐						
herpes simplex oralis		☐						
oesophageal herpes simplex		☐						
bronchitis	☐	☐	☐	☐	☐			
anorectal infection	☐	☐	☐	☐	☐			
cystitis	☐	☐	☐	☐	☐			
pyelonephritis	☐	☐	☐	☐	☐			
genital infection	☐	☐	☐	☐	☐			
skin infection	☐	☐	☐	☐	☐			
wound infection	☐	☐	☐	☐	☐			
phlebitis after needle puncture	☐	☐	☐	☐	☐			
fever of unknown origin					☐			
	☐	☐	☐	☐	☐			
	☐	☐	☐	☐	☐			
	☐	☐	☐	☐	☐			
	☐	☐	☐	☐	☐			
	☐	☐	☐	☐	☐			
	☐	☐	☐	☐	☐			
	☐	☐	☐	☐	☐			

*) caused by: B-bacteria; V-viruses; F-fungi; P-protozoa; UK-unknown

2.3 serological evidence of viral infection or preceding viral exposure

all no ☐, all unknown ☐, if so proceed to 3.5

Virus	Prior to Exposure yes, no, uk			After the Exposure yes, no, uk		
cytomegaly	☐	☐	☐	☐	☐	☐
Epstein-Barr	☐	☐	☐	☐	☐	☐
hepatitis-A	☐	☐	☐	☐	☐	☐
hepatitis-B	☐	☐	☐	☐	☐	☐
hepatitis-C	☐	☐	☐	☐	☐	☐
hepatitis-D	☐	☐	☐	☐	☐	☐
herpes simplex	☐	☐	☐	☐	☐	☐
HIV	☐	☐	☐	☐	☐	☐
varicella zoster	☐	☐	☐	☐	☐	☐
	☐	☐	☐	☐	☐	☐
	☐	☐	☐	☐	☐	☐

3.5   Radiation Induced Lesions of Gastrointestinal Tract

3.5.1   Diagnostic Procedures

all no ☐, all unknown ☐

1. endoscopy ....yes ☐, no ☐, unknown ☐, if yes please add xerocopy

2. conventional X-ray ....yes ☐, no ☐, unknown ☐, if yes please add xerocopy

3. biopsy..yes ☐, no ☐, unknown ☐, if yes please add xerocopy

4. others ....yes ☐, no ☐, unknown ☐, if yes please add xerocopy,

if yes, please specify ....

3.5.2   Faeces Analysis

yes ☐, no ☐, unknown ☐, if yes please add xerocopy

3.5.3   Radiation Mucositis

all no ☐, all unknown ☐

> ☞   The term "Begin" indicates the date and time of onset. The term "End" represents date and time of resolution of signs and symptoms of mucositis. The "Maximum" represents the date and time of onset of the most severe lesions. The degree of maximum severity of lesions should be noted in the column marked "degree".
>
> Please use the following score to indicate the severity of radiation mucositis:
>
> 1 - desquamate oedematous mucositis: oedema, nacre mucosae of tongue, gingivae, and buccae, with teeth prints and with desquamation of epithelium in form of white plaques, resembling candidosis;
>
> 2 - erosive mucositis: on ground of oedematous desquamation leading to erosions;
>
> 3 - ulcerative mucositis: there are deep defects of lamina muscularis mucosae
>
> 4 - necrotic mucositis: deep necrosis lamina muscularis mucosae with deep and extended oedema and severe pain

Site	yes	no	uk	Begin (Date & Time)	End (Date & Time)	Maximum (Date & Time)	Degree
lips	☐	☐	☐				
oral vestibule	☐	☐	☐				
sublingual space	☐	☐	☐				
soft palate	☐	☐	☐				
palatine tonsils	☐	☐	☐				
pharynx	☐	☐	☐				
hard palate, gums	☐	☐	☐				
back of tongue	☐	☐	☐				
radiation oesophagitis	☐	☐	☐				
infectious complications	☐	☐	☐				
	☐	☐	☐				

3.5.4   Acute Gastrointestinal Syndrome

all no ☐, all unknown ☐

Symptom/Sign	yes	no	uk	Begin (Date & Time)	End (Date & Time)	Maximum (Date & Time)	Degree
diarrhoea	☐	☐	☐				
disturbed gut passage: paralytic ileus	☐	☐	☐				
disturbed gut passage: mechanic ileus	☐	☐	☐				
pain	☐	☐	☐				
perforation	☐	☐	☐				
peritonitis	☐	☐	☐				
	☐	☐	☐				

3.5.5   Stool Characteristics

yes ☐, no ☐, unknown ☐, if yes please fill in the subsequent table

Date and Time	Frequency [# per day]	Volume [l/d]	Characteristic *

*)   Stool Characteristics

| constipation | cs | solid | sd | soft | sf | soft, watery | sfw | soft with blood | sfb |
| watery | wt | watery with blood | wtb | profuse | pf | profuse with blood | pfb |

3.6 Organs Especially Sensitive Under Certain Exposure Conditions

3.6.1 Lesions of Upper Respiratory Tract and Lung

1. diagnostic procedures ....all no ☐, all unknown ☐

1.1 blood-gas-analysis ....yes ☐, no ☐, unknown ☐, if yes please add xerocopy

1.2 conventional X-ray ....yes ☐, no ☐, unknown ☐, if yes please add xerocopy

1.3 CT ....yes ☐, no ☐, unknown ☐, if yes please add xerocopy

1.4 NMR ....yes ☐, no ☐, unknown ☐, if yes please add xerocopy

1.5 sonogram ....yes ☐, no ☐, unknown ☐, if yes please add xerocopy

1.6 bronchoscopy ....yes ☐, no ☐, unknown ☐, if yes please add xerocopy

1.7 others ....yes ☐, no ☐, unknown ☐, if yes please add xerocopy,

if yes, please specify ....

2. symptoms and signs of lesions of URT, lungs, and of adult respiratory distress syndrome (ARDS)

all no ☐, all unknown ☐

Symptom/Sign	yes	no	uk	Begin (Date & Time)	End (Date & Time)	Maximum (Date & Time)	Degree
postirradiative hyperaemia of URT	☐	☐	☐				
postirradiative erosion and ulcer of URT	☐	☐	☐				
cough	☐	☐	☐				
dyspnea (> 30/min)	☐	☐	☐				
hypoxaemia (art. blood only, PO < 70 mm Hg)	☐	☐	☐				
X-ray signs of ARDS	☐	☐	☐				
local pneumonia	☐	☐	☐				
interstitial diffuse pneumonitis	☐	☐	☐				
oedema of lungs	☐	☐	☐				
	☐	☐	☐				

3. laboratory data   yes ☐, no ☐, unknown ☐, if yes please continue

Blood Gas Analysis (1)

	Date and Time	Source of Blood art ven cap	pO_2 [mm Hg]	pCO_2 [mm Hg]	pH	Base Excess [mmol/l]	B.-Buffer [mmol/l]	Hb-O_2 [%]	Acid Buffer [mmol/l]
1		☐ ☐ ☐							
2		☐ ☐ ☐							
3		☐ ☐ ☐							
4		☐ ☐ ☐							
5		☐ ☐ ☐							
6		☐ ☐ ☐							
7		☐ ☐ ☐							
8		☐ ☐ ☐							
9		☐ ☐ ☐							
10		☐ ☐ ☐							
11		☐ ☐ ☐							
12		☐ ☐ ☐							
13		☐ ☐ ☐							
14		☐ ☐ ☐							
15		☐ ☐ ☐							
16		☐ ☐ ☐							
17		☐ ☐ ☐							
18		☐ ☐ ☐							
19		☐ ☐ ☐							
20		☐ ☐ ☐							
21		☐ ☐ ☐							
22		☐ ☐ ☐							
23		☐ ☐ ☐							
24		☐ ☐ ☐							
25		☐ ☐ ☐							
26		☐ ☐ ☐							
27		☐ ☐ ☐							
28		☐ ☐ ☐							
29		☐ ☐ ☐							
30		☐ ☐ ☐							

Blood Gas Analysis (1, right)

	SBC [%]	−HCO$_3$ [mmol/l]									
1											
2											
3											
4											
5											
6											
7											
8											
9											
10											
11											
12											
13											
14											
15											
16											
17											
18											
19											
20											
21											
22											
23											
24											
25											
26											
27											
28											
29											
30											

3.6.2   Lesions of the Thyroid Gland

1. diagnostic procedures..all no ☐, all unknown ☐

1.1 sonogram...yes ☐, no ☐, unknown ☐, if yes please add xerocopy

1.2 puncture ....yes ☐, no ☐, unknown ☐, if yes please add xerocopy

1.3 others ....yes ☐, no ☐, unknown ☐, if yes please add xerocopy,

   if yes, please specify...

2. clinical symptoms and signs   all no ☐, all unknown ☐

Symptom/Sign	yes	no	uk	Begin (Date & Time)	End (Date & Time)	Maximum (Date & Time)	Degree
myxedema	☐	☐	☐				
other signs related to hypothyroidism	☐	☐	☐				
	☐	☐	☐				
	☐	☐	☐				

3. laboratory data   yes ☐, no ☐, unknown ☐, if yes please continue

	Date and Time	^{131}J in Thyroid Gland [Bq]	Dose to Thyroid Gland [Sv]	TSH [mU/l]	T3 [µmol/l]	T4 [µmol/l]			
1									
2									
3									
4									
5									
6									
7									
8									
9									
10									

3.6.3   Pregnancy

yes ☐, no ☐, unknown ☐, if yes please fill in the subsequent table

week		fetal dose estimation [Sv]	
intrauterine death	yes ☐, no ☐, unknown ☐	if yes specify date [dd.mm.yyyy]	
abortus	yes ☐, no ☐, unknown ☐	if yes specify date [dd.mm.yyyy]	
delivery	yes ☐, no ☐, unknown ☐	if yes specify date [dd.mm.yyyy]	

3.7   Lesions of Other Organs

3.7.1   Lesions of the Kidneys

1. diagnostic procedures...all no ☐, all unknown ☐

1.1 sonogram...yes ☐, no ☐, unknown ☐, if yes please add xerocopy

1.2 conventional X-ray ....yes ☐, no ☐, unknown ☐, if yes please add xerocopy

1.3 CT ....yes ☐, no ☐, unknown ☐, if yes please add xerocopy

1.4 biopsy...yes ☐, no ☐, unknown ☐, if yes please add xerocopy

1.5 others ....yes ☐, no ☐, unknown ☐, if yes please add xerocopy,

if yes, please specify...

2. clinical symptoms and signs   all no ☐, all unknown ☐

Symptom/Sign	yes	no	uk	Begin (Date & Time)	End (Date & Time)	Maximum (Date & Time)	Degree
anuria	☐	☐	☐				
anuria requiring dialysis	☐	☐	☐				
arterial hypertension (BP >160/90)	☐	☐	☐				
creatinine level elevation (>130%N)	☐	☐	☐				
edema of face	☐	☐	☐				
hypertension requiring treatment	☐	☐	☐				
oliguria (100-500 ml/d)	☐	☐	☐				
polyuria	☐	☐	☐				
proteinuria (>1 %)	☐	☐	☐				
	☐	☐	☐				

3. urine analysis   yes ☐, no ☐, unknown ☐, if yes please continue

Urine Analysis (1, left)

	Date and Time	Glucose [mmol/l]	Uric Acid [mmol/l]	Creati-nine [mmol/l]	Total Protein [g/l]	Albumin [g/l]	Amylase (Urine) [U/l]	Na [mmol/l]	K [mmol/l]
1									
2									
3									
4									
5									
6									
7									
8									
9									
10									
11									
12									
13									
14									
15									
16									
17									
18									
19									
20									
21									
22									
23									
24									
25									
26									
27									
28									
29									
30									

Urine Analysis (1, right)

	Ca [mmol/l]	Chloride [mmol/l]	U-Phos-phorus [mmol/l]	Specific Gravity [#]	Osmola-rity [mOsm/l]	pH [#]	Amount of Urine [l/d]	WBC per Field [#]	RBC per Field [#]	Casts per Field [#]	
1											
2											
3											
4											
5											
6											
7											
8											
9											
10											
11											
12											
13											
14											
15											
16											
17											
18											
19											
20											
21											
22											
23											
24											
25											
26											
27											
28											
29											
30											

3.7.2   Lesions of the Liver

1. diagnostic procedures..all no ☐, all unknown ☐

1.1 sonogram..yes ☐, no ☐, unknown ☐, if yes please add xerocopy

1.2 CT ....yes ☐, no ☐, unknown ☐, if yes please add xerocopy

1.3 NMR ....yes ☐, no ☐, unknown ☐, if yes please add xerocopy

1.4 biopsy...yes ☐, no ☐, unknown ☐, if yes please add xerocopy

1.5 others ....yes ☐, no ☐, unknown ☐, if yes please add xerocopy,

if yes, please specify...

2. clinical symptoms and signs   all no ☐, all unknown ☐

Symptom/Sign	yes	no	uk	Begin (Date & Time)	End (Date & Time)	Maximum (Date & Time)	Degree
biochemical disorders	☐	☐	☐				
hepatic encephalopathy	☐	☐	☐				
hepatic venoocclusive disease (VOD)	☐	☐	☐				
hepatomegaly	☐	☐	☐				
ascites	☐	☐	☐				
hist. signs other than hepatitis and GvHD	☐	☐	☐				
jaundice	☐	☐	☐				
rapid gain of body weight	☐	☐	☐				
serological signs of viral hepatitis	☐	☐	☐				
viral transfusion hepatitis	☐	☐	☐				
	☐	☐	☐				

3.7.3   Evaluation of Male Reproductive Function

1. lesions of genital organs   all no ☐, all unknown ☐

Symptom/Sign	yes	no	uk	Begin (Date & Time)	End (Date & Time)	Maximum (Date & Time)	Degree
scrotal dermatitis	☐	☐	☐				
epilation of pubis	☐	☐	☐				
atrophy of testis	☐	☐	☐				
bioptical changes	☐	☐	☐				
	☐	☐	☐				

2. ejaculate evaluation   yes ☐, no ☐, unknown ☐, if yes please continue

Date and Time	Volume [ml]	Cell Count [Mega/l]	Normal Cells [%]	Mobility * n m imm	Spermatocytes [%]
				☐ ☐ ☐	
				☐ ☐ ☐	
				☐ ☐ ☐	
				☐ ☐ ☐	
				☐ ☐ ☐	

*)   Abbreviations used:
       normal mobility   n   medium mobility   m   immobile   imm

3.7.4   Evaluation of Female Reproductive Function

1. lesions of genital organs   all no ☐, all unknown ☐

Symptom/Sign	yes	no	uk	Begin (Date & Time)	End (Date & Time)	Maximum (Date & Time)	Degree
dermatitis	☐	☐	☐				
epilation of pubis	☐	☐	☐				
atrophy of ovaries	☐	☐	☐				
bioptical changes	☐	☐	☐				
	☐	☐	☐				

2. menstruation prior to exposure   yes ☐, no ☐, unknown ☐, if yes please continue

date of last menses before irradiation [dd.mm.yyyy]		menstruation recurred after irradiation	yes ☐, no ☐, unknown ☐
date of first menses after irradiation [dd.mm.yyyy]			

☞   See also chapter on Pregnancy

3.7.5   Lesions of Cardio-Vascular System

1. diagnostic procedures ....all no ☐, all unknown ☐

1.1 ECG ....yes ☐, no ☐, unknown ☐, if yes please add xerocopy

1.2 ergometric tests ....yes ☐, no ☐, unknown ☐, if yes please add xerocopy

1.3 echocardiography ....yes ☐, no ☐, unknown ☐, if yes please add xerocopy

1.4 conventional x-ray ....yes ☐, no ☐, unknown ☐, if yes please add xerocopy

1.5 biopsy...yes ☐, no ☐, unknown ☐, if yes please add xerocopy

1.5 others ....yes ☐, no ☐, unknown ☐, if yes please add xerocopy,

if yes, please specify..

2. disturbances of rhythm and conductivity   all no ☐, all unknown ☐

Symptom/Sign	yes	no	uk	Begin (Date & Time)	End (Date & Time)	Maximum (Date & Time)	Degree
supraventricular extrasystoles	☐	☐	☐				
ventricular extrasystoles	☐	☐	☐				
	☐	☐	☐				

3. toxic cardiomyopathy symptoms   all no ☐, all unknown ☐

Symptom/Sign	yes	no	uk	Begin (Date & Time)	End (Date & Time)	Maximum (Date & Time)	Degree
tachycardia discording with fever (>100-120/min)	☐	☐	☐				
muteness of cardiac tone	☐	☐	☐				
three tone rhythm	☐	☐	☐				
pre systolic gallop rhythm	☐	☐	☐				
dyspnea	☐	☐	☐				
cong. pulmonar signs (X-ray)	☐	☐	☐				
decrease of blood volume per minute	☐	☐	☐				
"specific" ECG changes	☐	☐	☐				
elevation of CV pressure	☐	☐	☐				
	☐	☐	☐				

4. general small vessels disease   all no ☐, all unknown ☐

Symptom/Sign	yes	no	uk	Begin (Date & Time)	End (Date & Time)	Maximum (Date & Time)	Degree
early edema of all tissues	☐	☐	☐				
severe hypotension	☐	☐	☐				
	☐	☐	☐				

3.7.6 General Physiological Parameters

yes ☐, no ☐, unknown ☐, if yes please fill in the subsequent table

	Date and Time	Weight [kg]	Blood Pressure [mm Hg]	Maximal Tempera- ture [° C]	Pulse [1/min]		
1							
2							
3							
4							
5							
6							
7							
8							
9							
10							
11							
12							
13							
14							
15							
16							
17							
18							
19							
20							
21							
22							
23							
24							
25							
26							
27							
28							
29							
30							

To continue, please make a list on your own by using this scheme and attach it to the questionnaire.

4.   Treatment and Drugs

4.1   Individual Radiation Protection Measures

4.1.1   Application of Personal Radiation Protectants during the Accident

all no ☐, all unknown ☐

Method	yes	no	uk	Begin (Date & Time)	End (Date & Time)
insulating clothes	☐	☐	☐		
mask, respirator	☐	☐	☐		
radio protective drugs	☐	☐	☐		
	☐	☐	☐		

4.1.2   Methods (Drugs) of Early Pathogenetical Treatment

all no ☐, all unknown ☐

Method	yes	no	uk	Begin (Date & Time)	End (Date & Time)
	☐	☐	☐		
	☐	☐	☐		
	☐	☐	☐		
	☐	☐	☐		

4.1.3   Decontamination Measures

all no ☐, all unknown ☐

Site	yes	no	uk	Begin (Date & Time)	End (Date & Time)
at the site of the accident	☐	☐	☐		
at the hospital	☐	☐	☐		
	☐	☐	☐		
	☐	☐	☐		

4.1.4 Decorporation Measures

all no ☐, all unknown ☐

Method	yes	no	uk	Begin (Date & Time)	End (Date & Time)
	☐	☐	☐		
	☐	☐	☐		
	☐	☐	☐		
	☐	☐	☐		

4.2 Physical Methods of Treatment

4.2.1 Hospitalisation and Protective Environment

all no ☐, all unknown ☐

Method	yes	no	uk	Begin (Date & Time)	End (Date & Time)	Site
outpatient care	☐	☐	☐			
hospitalisation	☐	☐	☐			
ordinary room	☐	☐	☐			
reversed isolation	☐	☐	☐			
high press. room, filt. air incld. HEPA, laminar air flow	☐	☐	☐			
sterile food	☐	☐	☐			
total parenteral	☐	☐	☐			
	☐	☐	☐			

4.2.2 Locally Reversed Isolation for Burn Treatment

all no ☐, all unknown ☐

Isolated part of the body ‡	Begin (Date & Time)	End (Date & Time)	Type of Isolation

‡) For coding please use numbers of chapter 6.2 to 6.4

4.3 Substituting Therapy by Blood and Blood Products

yes ☐, no ☐, unknown ☐, if yes, please continue with 4.3.1, otherwise please proceed to 4.4

4.3.1 Irradiation of Blood and Blood Products

yes ☐, no ☐, unknown ☐, if yes please give the irradiation dose [Gy] _____

4.3.2 Blood Groups and Alloimmunisation

1. lymphocytotoxicity against random donors   yes ☐, no ☐, unknown ☐, if yes please continue

Date and Time	% Positive Reactions	No. of Evaluated Random Donors

2. blood typing   yes ☐, no ☐, unknown ☐, if yes please continue

Blood Groups

ABO-System

Group	All. 1	All. 2	Comment
A	☐	☐	
A1	☐	☐	
A2	☐	☐	
B	☐	☐	
0	☐	☐	

MNSs-System

Group	All. 1	All. 2	Comment
M	☐	☐	
N	☐	☐	
S	☐	☐	
s	☐	☐	

Kell-System

Kell pos   ☐ Kell neg   ☐,
if more detailed information is available please continue

Group	All. 1	All. 2	Comment
K	☐	☐	
k	☐	☐	
kp^a	☐	☐	
kb^b	☐	☐	
ls^a	☐	☐	
ls^b	☐	☐	

Rhesus-System

Rhesus pos ☐ Rhesus neg ☐,

if more detailed information is available please continue

Group	All. 1	All. 2	Comment
C	☐	☐	
C^w	☐	☐	
c	☐	☐	
D	☐	☐	
D^u	☐	☐	
d	☐	☐	
E	☐	☐	
e	☐	☐	

Lewis-System

Group	All. 1	All. 2	Comment
Le^a	☐	☐	
Le^b	☐	☐	

Lutheran-System

Group	All. 1	All. 2	Comment
Lu^a	☐	☐	
Lu^b	☐	☐	

Kidd-System

Group	All. 1	All. 2	Comment
Ik^a	☐	☐	
Ik^b	☐	☐	

Duffy System

Fy(a)pos ☐ Fy(b)neg ☐,

if more detailed information is available please continue

Group	All. 1	All. 2	Comment
Fy^a	☐	☐	
Fy^b	☐	☐	
Fy	☐	☐	

HLA-System

Group	Allele 1	Allele 2
A		
B		
C		
DR		
DQ		
DP		

4.3.3 Whole Blood Transfusions

yes ☐, no ☐, unknown ☐, if yes please fill in the subsequent table

Date and Time	Quantity [ml]	Quantity [Units*]	Transfusion Reaction
			yes ☐, no ☐, uk ☐
			yes ☐, no ☐, uk ☐
			yes ☐, no ☐, uk ☐
			yes ☐, no ☐, uk ☐
			yes ☐, no ☐, uk ☐
			yes ☐, no ☐, uk ☐
			yes ☐, no ☐, uk ☐
			yes ☐, no ☐, uk ☐
			yes ☐, no ☐, uk ☐
			yes ☐, no ☐, uk ☐

*)   one standard whole blood unit, i. e., 400 - 450 ml

4.3.4 Red Blood Cell Transfusions

yes ☐, no ☐, unknown ☐, if yes please fill in the subsequent table

Date and Time*	Quantity [ml]	Quantity [Units*]	Transfusion Reaction
			yes ☐, no ☐, uk ☐
			yes ☐, no ☐, uk ☐
			yes ☐, no ☐, uk ☐
			yes ☐, no ☐, uk ☐
			yes ☐, no ☐, uk ☐
			yes ☐, no ☐, uk ☐
			yes ☐, no ☐, uk ☐
			yes ☐, no ☐, uk ☐
			yes ☐, no ☐, uk ☐
			yes ☐, no ☐, uk ☐

*)   if necessary please continue by adding a xerocopy

*)   amount of cells derived from one standard whole blood unit, i. e., 400 - 450 ml

4.3.5 Platelet Transfusions and Thrombocytapheresis

1. platelet transfusion   yes ☐, no ☐, unknown ☐, if yes please fill in the subsequent table

Date and Time*	Quantity [100 Giga]	Quantity [Units*]	Fresh° auto allo	Cryopre-served° auto allo	Donor • sg pld	ABO matched y no uk	HLA matched y no uk	Transf. Reaction y no uk
			☐ ☐	☐ ☐	☐ ☐	☐☐☐	☐☐☐	☐☐☐
			☐ ☐	☐ ☐	☐ ☐	☐☐☐	☐☐☐	☐☐☐
			☐ ☐	☐ ☐	☐ ☐	☐☐☐	☐☐☐	☐☐☐
			☐ ☐	☐ ☐	☐ ☐	☐☐☐	☐☐☐	☐☐☐
			☐ ☐	☐ ☐	☐ ☐	☐☐☐	☐☐☐	☐☐☐
			☐ ☐	☐ ☐	☐ ☐	☐☐☐	☐☐☐	☐☐☐
			☐ ☐	☐ ☐	☐ ☐	☐☐☐	☐☐☐	☐☐☐
			☐ ☐	☐ ☐	☐ ☐	☐☐☐	☐☐☐	☐☐☐
			☐ ☐	☐ ☐	☐ ☐	☐☐☐	☐☐☐	☐☐☐
			☐ ☐	☐ ☐	☐ ☐	☐☐☐	☐☐☐	☐☐☐

*)   if necessary please continue by adding a xerocopy

*)   amount of cells derived from one standard whole blood unit, i. e., 400 - 450 ml

     Abbreviations used

°)   autologous   auto   allogeneic   allo   •)   single donor   sg   pooled   pld

2. thrombocytapheresis (TAPH)   yes ☐, no ☐, unknown ☐, if yes please continue

Date and Time*	Blood Volume processed [l]	Gain of Platelets [100 Giga]	Gain of Platelets [Units*]

*) if necessary please continue by adding a xerocopy

*) amount of cells derived from one standard whole blood unit, i. e., 400 - 450 ml

4.3.6   White Blood Cell Transfusions

yes ☐, no ☐, unknown ☐, if yes please fill in the subsequent table

Date and Time*	Volume [ml]	Transf. WBC [Giga]	Transf. Gra-nulocytes [Giga]	Transf. Mo-nonuclear Cells [Giga]	Donor +) N CML	Transfus. Reaction yes no uk
					☐ ☐	☐ ☐ ☐
					☐ ☐	☐ ☐ ☐
					☐ ☐	☐ ☐ ☐
					☐ ☐	☐ ☐ ☐
					☐ ☐	☐ ☐ ☐
					☐ ☐	☐ ☐ ☐
					☐ ☐	☐ ☐ ☐
					☐ ☐	☐ ☐ ☐
					☐ ☐	☐ ☐ ☐
					☐ ☐	☐ ☐ ☐

*) if necessary please continue by adding a xerocopy

+) Abbreviations used

regular donor   N   patient with chronic myeloid leukemia as donor   CML

4.3.7   Plasma Transfusions and Plasmapheresis

1. plasma transfusions   yes ☐, no ☐, unknown ☐, if yes please continue

Date and Time*	Transfused Volume [l]	Quantity [Units*]	Type of Plasma+	Transfusion Reaction
			ntv ☐, cp ☐, dr ☐	yes ☐, no ☐, uk ☐
			ntv ☐, cp ☐, dr ☐	yes ☐, no ☐, uk ☐
			ntv ☐, cp ☐, dr ☐	yes ☐, no ☐, uk ☐
			ntv ☐, cp ☐, dr ☐	yes ☐, no ☐, uk ☐
			ntv ☐, cp ☐, dr ☐	yes ☐, no ☐, uk ☐
			ntv ☐, cp ☐, dr ☐	yes ☐, no ☐, uk ☐
			ntv ☐, cp ☐, dr ☐	yes ☐, no ☐, uk ☐
			ntv ☐, cp ☐, dr ☐	yes ☐, no ☐, uk ☐
			ntv ☐, cp ☐, dr ☐	yes ☐, no ☐, uk ☐
			ntv ☐, cp ☐, dr ☐	yes ☐, no ☐, uk ☐

*)   if necessary please continue by adding a xerocopy

*)   amount of plasma derived from one standard whole blood unit, i. e., 400 - 450 ml

+)   Abbreviations used

      native   ntv   cryopreserved   cp   dry   dr

2. plasmapheresis (PAPH)   yes ☐, no ☐, unknown ☐, if yes please fill in the subsequent table

Date and Time*	Blood Volume processed [l]	Plasma Volume discarded [l]	Total Infused Volume [l]	Plasma Volume Infused [l]	Saline Volume Infused [l]	10% Albumin Sol. Volume Infused [l]]

*)   if necessary please continue

4.3.8 Albumin Solution Infusions, Gamma Globulin Substitution and Other Blood Components

yes ☐, no ☐, unknown ☐, if yes please be sure to enter the data required in table 4.4.

The appropriate form of entry applies also.

4.4 Drugs

yes ☐, no ☐, unknown ☐, if yes, please continue with 4.4.1, if no or unknown please proceed to 4.5

☞ Please insert in the subsequent table 4.4.1 the names of the drugs applying the rules listed below.

The drugs can be written down in arbitrary order. When there is a change of daily dose, signature, or form of administration please use a new line. If necessary, please add a xerocopy of the prescription of pharmaceuticals not provided by pharmaceutical industry

---

Instructions for Use

INN-Name	INN means International Nonproprietory Names for Pharmaceutical Substances published by WHO. As a reference source you are, in doubt, requested to refer to the Index Nominum™. In the case of drugs composed of multiple or ill-defined chemical compounds please give the trade mark. This should be indicated by an asterisk at the end of the name. If a speciality is supplied in different concentrations you are requested to indicate the concentration in this column too, e.g. *glucose 5%*.
Daily Dose [g]	If the dose can be given as a mass it should be expressed as "g". This implies that fractions of a gram, e. g., milli-gram should be expressed as *ne-3* g. For correct transformation of the relevant units please to refer to the annex 8.3.
Daily Dose [iU]	If the dose can be expressed in international units it should be given as "iU". This implies that fractions or the multiple of an iU, e. g., Mega-iU should be expressed as *ne6* iU. For correct transformation of the relevant units please refer to the annex 8.3.
Daily Dose [ml]	In case the dose can be given as a volume it should be expressed as "ml".
Signature	The signature should expressed as number of administrations per number of days. If, for example a drug is applied three times per day, the entry will read 3/d. If there is on the other hand only 1 administration every other day the entry will thus read 1/2d.
Form of Administration	The form of administration should be coded as outlined below. If you want to express an *i. v. administration lasting for 6 hours*, you may enter *iv 6 h*. For a *continuous intrathecal* application please write *it 24 h*. If no dosage is available at all please include in this row the number of tablets etc. administered per day. If no suitable abbreviation is given below, please use free-text statements.
Begin/End of Administration	In most cases the use of date is sufficient. Time should only be given if and where appropriate

Abbreviations Used:

oral	o	inhaled	inh	eye	ey
rectal	r	external	ext	upper respiratory tract	URT
intravenous	iv	drop	dr	skin	sk
intramuscular	im	ointment	oi	others	ot
intrathecal	it	washing	wa	hour	h
subcutaneous	sc	mouth	mo	minute	m
intracutaneous	ic	wound	wo	second	s

Administered Drugs (1, left)

	INN-Name	Daily Dose [g]	Daily Dose [iU]	Daily Dose [ml]
1				
2				
3				
4				
5				
6				
7				
8				
9				
10				
11				
12				
13				
14				
15				
16				
17				
18				
19				
20				
21				
22				
23				
24				
25				
26				
27				
28				
29				
30				

Administered Drugs (1, right)

	Signature	Form of Administration[*]	Begin of Administration [Date and Time]	End of Administration [Date and Time]
1				
2				
3				
4				
5				
6				
7				
8				
9				
10				
11				
12				
13				
14				
15				
16				
17				
18				
19				
20				
21				
22				
23				
24				
25				
26				
27				
28				
29				
30				

[*]if possible please use abbreviations as explained above (see 4.4)

Administered Drugs (2, left)*

	INN-Name	Daily Dose [g]	Daily Dose [iU]	Daily Dose [ml]
31				
32				
33				
34				
35				
36				
37				
38				
39				
40				
41				
42				
43				
44				
45				
46				
47				
48				
49				
50				
51				
52				
53				
54				
55				
56				
57				
58				
59				
60				

*)   if necessary please continue by adding a xerocopy

Administered Drugs (2, right)

	Signature	Form of Administration	Begin of Administration [Date and Time]	End of Administration [Date and Time]
31				
32				
33				
34				
35				
36				
37				
38				
39				
40				
41				
42				
43				
44				
45				
46				
47				
48				
49				
50				
51				
52				
53				
54				
55				
56				
57				
58				
59				
60				

*if possible please use abbreviations as explained above (see 4.4)

4.5   Haemostimulators

4.5.1   Myelopoietic Growth Factors

yes ☐, no ☐, unknown ☐, if yes please continue

Name of Drugs (preferably INN)	

☞   Please be sure to enter the data required in table 4.4. The appropriate form of entry applies to growth factors also.

4.5.2   Other Growth Factors

yes ☐, no ☐, unknown ☐, if yes please continue

Name of Drugs (preferably INN)	

☞   Please be sure to enter the data required in table 4.4. The appropriate form of entry applies to growth factors also.

4.5.3   Drugs as Leucostimulators

yes ☐, no ☐, unknown ☐, if yes please continue

Name of Drugs (preferably INN)	

☞   Please be sure to enter the data required in table 4.4. The appropriate form of entry applies to growth factors also.

4.6   Haemopoietic Stem Cell Transplantation

☐ performed, please complete chapter 7

☐ planned but not performed, please complete chapter 7

☐ not planned

☐ unknown

5.   Clinical Status at the Time of Reporting

5.1   Survival Status

5.1.1   General Information on the Survival Status

Date and Time of Reporting [dd.mm.yyyy] [hh:mm]		Patient is still alive	yes ☐ no ☐ follow-up lost ☐

5.1.2   Loss of Follow-Up

Last date the patient has been known to be alive [dd.mm.yyyy]	

5.1.3   Death of Patient

Date and Time of Death [dd.mm.yyyy] [hh:mm]		A Necropsy was Performed	yes ☐, no ☐, unknown ☐
Extramedullary Haemopoiesis	yes ☐, no ☐, unknown ☐	if yes specify	

5.1.4   Causes of Death

Causal Factors	Primary Cause *)	Contribu-ting Cause	Comment	ICD-No.
radiation induced brain damage	☐	☐		
radiation induced skin damage	☐	☐		
radiation induced gut damage	☐	☐		
interstitial pneumonitis	☐	☐		
other pneumonia	☐	☐		
bacterial infection	☐	☐		
viral infection	☐	☐		
fungal infection	☐	☐		
protozoal infection	☐	☐		
unclassified infection	☐	☐		
adult respiratory distress syndrome	☐	☐		
liver failure	☐	☐		
kidney failure	☐	☐		
heart failure	☐	☐		
disseminated intravascular coagulation	☐	☐		
veno-occlusive disease	☐	☐		
haemorrhage	☐	☐		
acute or chronic GvHD	☐	☐		
	☐	☐		
	☐	☐		

*)   Please do not use more than one primary cause as the cause of death

5.2   Clinical Status

5.2.1   Time of Evaluation

If differing from 5.1.1 please give date [dd.mm.yyyy]	

5.2.2   Radiation Related Persisting Haemopoietic Disorders

yes ☐, no ☐, unknown ☐, if yes please fill in the subsequent table

Diagnosis	ICD-No.

5.2.3   Other Persisting Haemopoietic Disorders

yes ☐, no ☐, unknown ☐, if yes please fill in the subsequent table

Diagnosis	ICD-No.

5.2.4 Radiation Related Persisting Lesions of Skin and Underlying Tissue

yes ☐, no ☐, unknown ☐, if yes please fill in the subsequent table

Diagnosis	ICD-No.

5.2.5 Other Persisting Lesions of Skin and Underlying Tissue

yes ☐, no ☐, unknown ☐, if yes please fill in the subsequent table

Diagnosis	ICD-No.

5.2.6 Radiation Related Persisting Lesions of Other Organs

yes ☐, no ☐, unknown ☐, if yes please fill in the subsequent table

Organ	Diagnosis	ICD-No.
brain and CNS		
lung		
eyes		
liver		
kidney		
GIT		

5.2.7   Additional Persisting Lesions of Other Organs

yes ☐, no ☐, unknown ☐, if yes please fill in the subsequent table

Organ	Diagnosis	ICD-No.
brain and CNS		
lung		
eyes		
liver		
kidney		
GIT		

5.3   Functional Status

5.3.1   Time of Evaluation

If differing from 5.1.1 please give date [dd.mm.yyyy]	

5.3.2   Karnofsky Performance Score

☞ For further explanation see annex 8.4

Percentage [%]	

5.3.3   Rehabilitation

1.   children > 6 ys. of age

patient currently attends school	yes ☐, no ☐, unknown ☐	full-time	yes ☐, no ☐, unknown ☐
part-time	yes ☐, no ☐, unknown ☐	date of return to school [dd.mm.yyyy]	

2.   adults > 20 ys. of age

patient resumed work	yes ☐, no ☐, unknown ☐	full-time	yes ☐, no ☐, unknown ☐
part-time	yes ☐, no ☐, unknown ☐	date of return to work [dd.mm.yyyy]	

6.   Skin Burns

6.1   Burn Score

The following five grade ordinary scale should be used for table 6.5

1. Phase of injury

0.0	no signs of skin burns (normal skin)
0.5	mild erythema
1.0	red (arterial) erythema
1.5	blue (veno-congestive) erythema (+ skin edema, + subcutaneous fat oedema) with transformation in pigmentation
2.0	moistening epidermitis (small, superficial, intraepidermal blisters)
2.5	blisters (gross, tension, dermo-epidermal)
3.0	erosions (no epidermis, no necrosis of derma)
3.5	ulcers (no epidermis, some degree derma lost)
4.0	necrosis of all skin layers
4.5	necrosis of skin and subcutaneous fat tissue
5.0	necrosis of skin, subcutaneous fat tissue, and underlying tissues

2. Phase of stability and recovery

-4.0-5.0	persisting necroses
-3.5	beginning of marginal epithelialisation of ulcers
-3.0	marked marginal epithelialisation of ulcers and erosions: >10-50% their surface
-2.5	marked marginal epithelialisation of ulcers and erosions: > 50% their surface
-2.0	almost complete reepithelialisation of ulcers and erosions
-1.5	complete epithelialisation of ulcer and erosions
-1.0	atrophic epidermis and dermal scars after ulcer, erosions and dry desquamation after pigmentation
-0.5	almost normal appearance of skin (after 1.0 or 1.5 in injury phase)
-0.0	normal skin (usually after 1.0-2.0)

6.2   Localisation Coding - Total Body, Head, Neck and Upper Trunk

Part	Subpart	Region	Subregion		Description
0					Total Body
1					Head
	1L				- left side
		1L1			-- Ear (left)
	1R				-right side
		1R1			-- Ear (right)
	1F				- front
		1F1			-- Eyes
			1F1L		--- Eye (left)
			1F1R		--- Eye (right
		1F2			-- Nose
		1F3			-- Mouth
	1B				- back
	1T				- top
2					Neck
	2L				
	2R				
	2F				
	2B				
3					Upper Trunk
	3L				
		3L1	3L1B/3L1F		-- Left Axilla
	3R				
		3R1	3R1B/3R1F		-- Right Axilla
	3F				- front
		3F1			-- quadrant upper right
		3F2			-- quadrant upper left
		3F3			-- quadrant lower left
		3F4			-- quadrant lower right
	3B				
		3B1			-- quadrant upper left
		3B2			-- quadrant upper right
		3B3			-- quadrant lower right
		3B4			-- quadrant lower left

6.3　Localisation Coding - Arms, Lower Trunk

Part	Subpart	Region	Subregion		Description
4					Arm
	4L				- Arm (left)
		4L1			-- upper arm proximal 3rd + shoulder
			4L1 L/R/F/B		
		4L2			-- upper arm medial 3rd + distal 3rd
			4L2 L/R/F/B		
		4L3			-- elbow
			4L3 L/R/F/B		
		4L4			-- forearm
			4L4 L/R/F/B		
		4L5			-- wrist
			4L5 L/R/F/B		
		4L6			-- hand (except fingers, thenar group)
			4L6L		
			4L6R		
			4L6F	4L6F L/R	--- palm
			4L6B	4L6B L/R	--- volar region
		4L7			-- fingers
			4L7.1	4L7.1 L/R/F/B	--- finger I + thenar group
			4L7.2	4L7.2 L/R/F/B	--- finger II
			4L7.3	4L7.3 L/R/F/B	--- finger III
			4L7.4	4L7.4 L/R/F/B	--- finger IV
			4L7.5	4L7.5 L/R/F/B	--- finger V
	4R				- Arm (right)
		4R1			-- upper arm proximal 3rd + shoulder
			4R1 L/R/F/B		
		4R2			-- upper arm medial 3rd + distal 3rd
			4R2 L/R/F/B		
		4R3			-- elbow
			4R3 L/R/F/B		
		4R4			-- forearm
			4R4 L/R/F/B		
		4R5			-- wrist
			4R5 L/R/F/B		
		4R6			-- hand (except fingers, thenar group)
			4R6L		
			4R6R		
			4R6F	4R6F L/R	--- palm
			4R6B	4R6B L/R	--- volar region
		4R7			-- fingers
			4R7.1	4R7.1 L/R/F/B	--- finger I + thenar group
			4R7.2	4R7.2 L/R/F/B	--- finger II
			4R7.3	4R7.3 L/R/F/B	--- finger III
			4R7.4	4R7.4 L/R/F/B	--- finger IV
			4R7.5	4R7.5 L/R/F/B	--- finger V
5					Lower Trunk
	5L				
	5R				
	5F				
		5F1			-- quadrant upper right
		5F2			-- quadrant upper left
		5F3			-- quadrant lower left
		5F4			-- quadrant lower right
	5B				
		5B1			-- quadrant upper left
		5B2			-- quadrant upper right
		5B3			-- quadrant lower right
		5B4			-- quadrant lower left

6.4   Localisation Coding - Lower Trunk, Legs

Part	Subpart	Region	Subregion		Description
6					Regio Pudenda, Perineum, Buttocks
	6F				- Regio Pudenda + Ext. Genital Organs
		6F1	6F1L/R		-- Regio Pudenda
		6F2	6F2L/R		-- External Genital Organs
		6F3	6F3L/R		-- Perineum
	6B				- Anal Region
		6B1	6B1L/R		-- Rima Ani
		6B2	6B2L/R		-- Anus
	6L				- Buttock (left)
		6L1			-- quadrant upper front
		6L2			-- quadrant upper back
		6L3			-- quadrant lower back
		6L4			-- quadrant lower front
	6R				- Buttock (right)
		6R1			-- quadrant upper front
		6R2			-- quadrant upper back
		6R3			-- quadrant lower back
		6R4			-- quadrant lower front
7					Leg
	7L				- Leg (left)
		7L1			-- thigh proximal 3rd
			7L1 L/R/F/B		
		7L2			-- thigh medial 3rd + thigh distal 3rd
			7L2 L/R/F/B		
		7L3			-- knee + knee pit
			7L3 L/R/F/B		
		7L4			-- shank
			7L4 L/R/F/B		
		7L5			-- ankle
			7L5 L/R/F/B		
		7L6			-- foot (except toes, thenar group)
			7L6L		
			7L6R		
			7L6F	7L6F L/R	--- sole
			7L6B	7L6B L/R	--- tarsal region
		7L7			-- fingers
			7L7.1	7L7.1 L/R/F/B	--- finger I + thenar group
			7L7.2	7L7.2 L/R/F/B	--- finger II
			7L7.3	7L7.3 L/R/F/B	--- finger III
			7L7.4	7L7.4 L/R/F/B	--- finger IV
			7L7.5	7L7.5 L/R/F/B	--- finger V
	7R				- Leg (right)
		7R1			-- thigh proximal 3rd
			7R1 L/R/F/B		
		7R2			-- thigh medial 3rd + thigh distal 3rd
			7R2 L/R/F/B		
		7R3			-- knee + knee pit
			7R3 L/R/F/B		
		7R4			-- shank
			7R4 L/R/F/B		
		7R5			-- ankle
			7R5 L/R/F/B		
		7R6			-- foot (except toes, thenar group)
			7R6L		
			7R6R		
			7R6F	7R6F L/R	--- sole
			7R6B	7R6B L/R	--- tarsal region
		7R7			-- fingers
			7R7.1	7R7.1 L/R/F/B	--- finger I + thenar group
			7R7.2	7R7.2 L/R/F/B	--- finger II
			7R7.3	7R7.3 L/R/F/B	--- finger III
			7R7.4	7R7.4 L/R/F/B	--- finger IV
			7R7.5	7R7.5 L/R/F/B	--- finger V

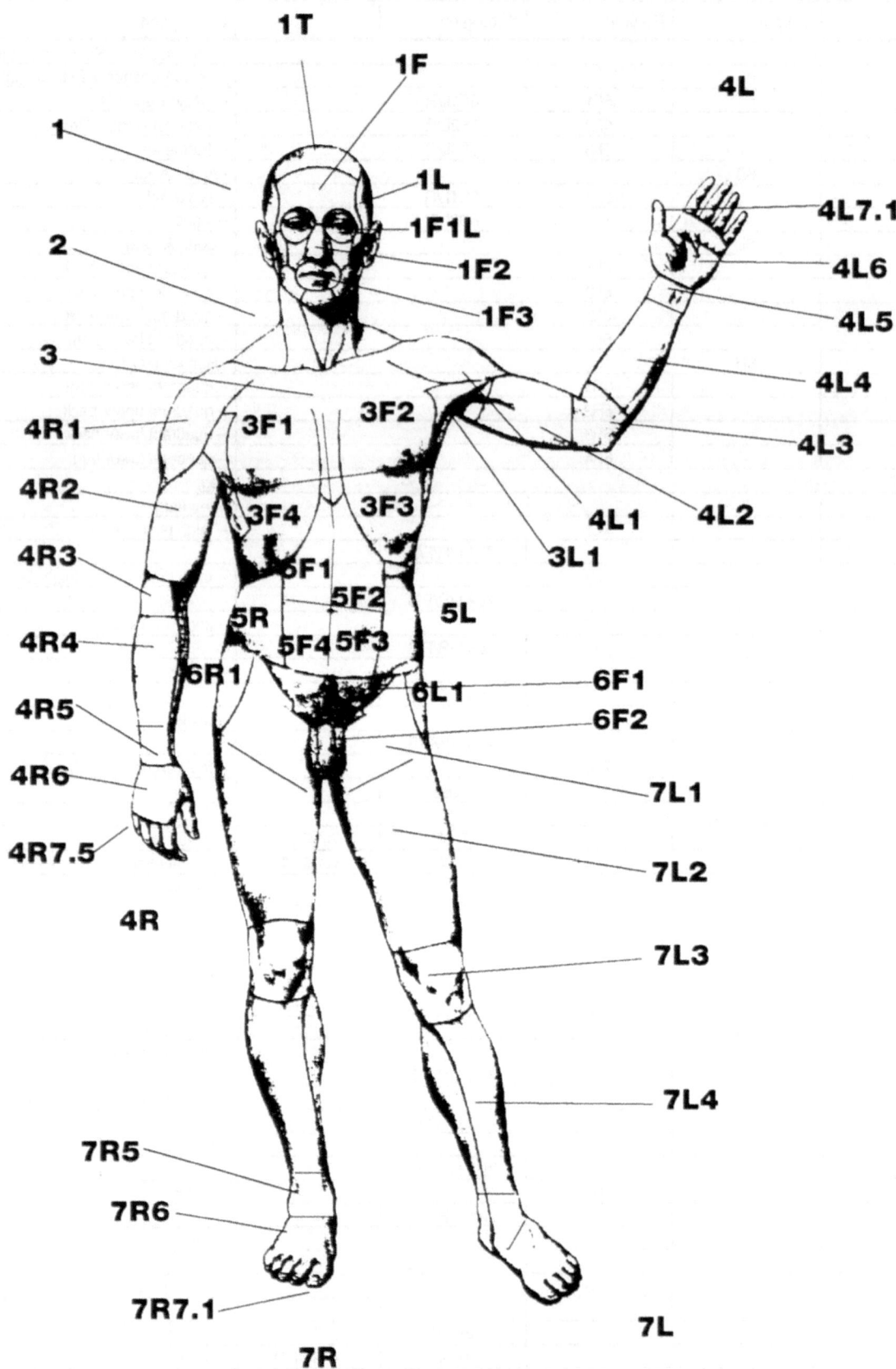

Human Body - Anterior View
(modified from Sobotta/Becher)

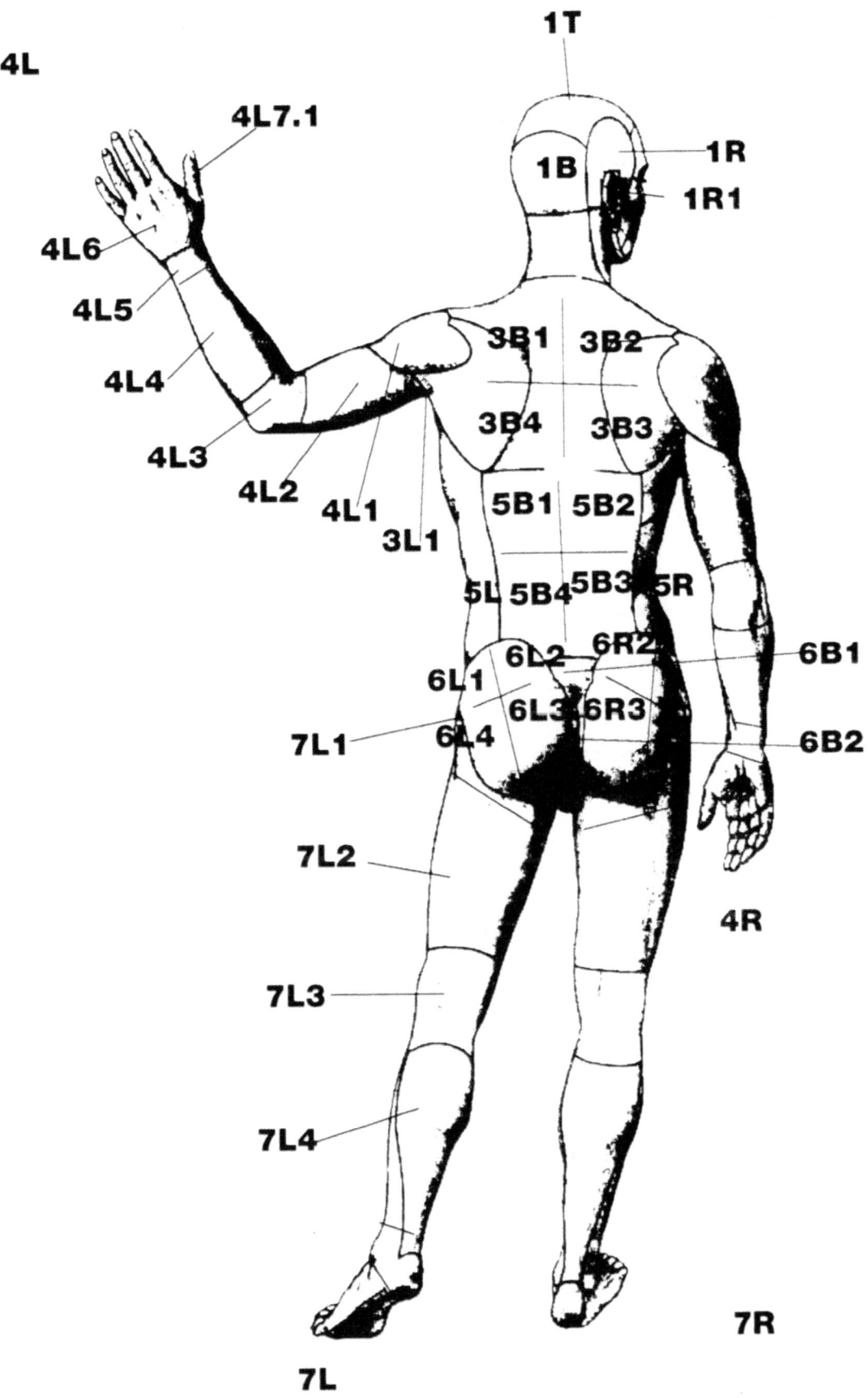

Human Body - Posterior View
(modified from Sobotta/Becher)

6.5   Skin Burns

Date and Time	Localisation (see 6.2)	Degree (see 6.1)	Involv. Surface [% body surface]	Involved Surface [cm²]

7. Haematopoietic Stem Cell Transplantation

7.1 Source of Stem Cells

bone marrow	yes ☐, no ☐, unknown ☐	peripheral blood	yes ☐, no ☐, unknown ☐
others	yes ☐, no ☐, unknown ☐	if yes specify	

7.2 Type of Transplantation

autologous	yes ☐, no ☐, unknown ☐	cryopres. agent if yes specify	
temperature of the cryopreservation [°C]			
allogeneic	yes ☐, no ☐, unknown ☐		
if yes specify			

7.3 Histocompatibility Tests for Allogeneic Transplantation

7.3.1 Typing

yes ☐, no ☐, unknown ☐, if yes please fill in the subsequent tables

1. donor

ABO-System

Group	All. 1	All. 2	Comment
A	☐	☐	
A1	☐	☐	
A2	☐	☐	
B	☐	☐	
0	☐	☐	

HLA-System

Group	All. 1	All. 2
A		
B		
C		
DR		
DQ		
DP		

2. mother

ABO-System

Group	All. 1	All. 2	Comment
A	☐	☐	
A1	☐	☐	
A2	☐	☐	
B	☐	☐	
0	☐	☐	

HLA-System

Group	All. 1	All. 2
A		
B		
C		
DR		
DQ		
DP		

3. father

ABO-System

Group	All. 1	All. 2	Comment
A	☐	☐	
A1	☐	☐	
A2	☐	☐	
B	☐	☐	
0	☐	☐	

HLA-System

Group	All. 1	All. 2
A		
B		
C		
DR		
DQ		
DP		

7.3.2 Donor and Recipient Cells Were Tested for Matching

matching (reciprocal non stimulation) in mixed leukocyte test	yes ☐, no ☐, unknown ☐	recipient cells responded to donor cells	yes ☐, no ☐, unknown ☐
donor cells responded to recipient cells	yes ☐, no ☐, unknown ☐		

7.4 Donor Information

7.4.1 Donor's Demographical Data

family name	
given name	

sex	male ☐	female ☐

age at the time of the accident [yyy]		Date of birth [dd.mm.yyyy]	

7.4.2 Donor Relationship and Alloimmunisation History

sibling	yes ☐, no ☐, unknown ☐	fraternal twin	yes ☐, no ☐, unknown ☐
identical twin	yes ☐, no ☐, unknown ☐	parent	yes ☐, no ☐, unknown ☐
child	yes ☐, no ☐, unknown ☐	otherly related	yes ☐, no ☐, unknown ☐
please specify		unrelated	yes ☐, no ☐, unknown ☐
donor had previous pregnancy	yes ☐, no ☐, unknown ☐	total number of pregnancies	
total number of male offspring			
donor had previous transfusion	yes ☐, no ☐, unknown ☐	total number of transfusion	

7.4.3 Donor had Serological Evidence of Previous Viral Exposure or Infection

all no ☐, all unknown ☐

Virus	yes, no, uk
cytomegaly	☐ ☐ ☐
Epstein-Barr	☐ ☐ ☐
hepatitis-A	☐ ☐ ☐
hepatitis-B	☐ ☐ ☐
hepatitis-C	☐ ☐ ☐
hepatitis-D	☐ ☐ ☐
herpes simplex	☐ ☐ ☐
varicella zoster	☐ ☐ ☐
HIV	☐ ☐ ☐

7.5 Transplant Manoeuvre

7.5.1 Conditioning Therapy prior to Stem Cell Therapy

supplement. irradi-ation, please specify	
drugs	yes ☐, no ☐, unknown ☐
date of transplant [dd.mm.yyyy]	nucleated cell dose [x10^8/kg]

7.5.2 Cells Were Manipulated or Concentrated in vitro

mechanical cell separator	yes ☐, no ☐, unknown ☐	Ficoll-Hypaque	yes ☐, no ☐, unknown ☐
starch gel sedimentation	yes ☐, no ☐, unknown ☐	other (do not include T-cell depletion)	yes ☐, no ☐, unknown ☐
specify			
total dose of T-cells [x10^5/kg]		no. of infused pro-genitors was tested	yes ☐, no ☐, unknown ☐
CFU-GM admin-istered [x10^3/kg]		CFU-GEMM [x10^3/kg]	
CFU-E [x10^3/kg]		BFU-E [x10^3/kg]	
boost application	yes ☐, no ☐, unknown ☐	date of boost [dd.mm.yyyy]	
nucleated cell dose [x10^8/kg]		boost was T-cell depleted	yes ☐, no ☐, unknown ☐

7.6 Drugs to Prevent Acute Graft-versus-Host Disease (GvHD)

yes ☐, no ☐, unknown ☐, if yes please be sure to enter the data required in table 4.4. The appropriate form of entry applies to these preventive measures also.

7.7 In vitro and in vivo Removal of Donor T Cells to Prevent GvHD

yes ☐, no ☐, unknown ☐, if yes please fill in the subsequent table

Measure of T-Cell Removal	Specification
antibody	
complement	
toxin	
magnetic beads	
lectin	
SRBC rossetting	
drug	
elution	
density gradient	

7.8 Evidence for Haemopoietic Engraftment

yes ☐, no ☐, unknown ☐, if yes please fill in the subsequent table

Marker	Date and Time of Measurement	Host [%]	Donor [%]
donor sex or other chromosome marker, specify below			
donor RBC or WBC marker, please specify below			
restriction fragment polymorphism, please specify below			
other methods			

7.9 Overall Evaluation of Engraftment

no engraftment	yes ☐, no ☐, unknown ☐	uncertain engraftment	yes ☐, no ☐, unknown ☐
loss of graft due to graft rejection	yes ☐, no ☐, unknown ☐	date of loss [dd.mm.yyyy]	
loss of graft due to septicaemia	yes ☐, no ☐, unknown ☐	date of loss [dd.mm.yyyy]	
loss of graft due to myelotoxic drugs	yes ☐, no ☐, unknown ☐	date of loss [dd.mm.yyyy]	
loss of graft due to other reasons	yes ☐, no ☐, unknown ☐	date of loss [dd.mm.yyyy]	
stable engraftment	yes ☐, no ☐, unknown ☐	date of engraftment [dd.mm.yyyy]	
autologous recovery of haemopoiesis	yes ☐, no ☐, unknown ☐	date of recovery [dd.mm.yyyy]	

7.10 Graft-versus-Host Disease

all no ☐, all unknown ☐

GvHD*)	yes	no	uk	Begin	End	Maximum	Degree
acute GvHD	☐	☐	☐				
chronic GvHD	☐	☐	☐				
dermal signs of acute GvHD	☐	☐	☐				
dermal signs of chronic GvHD	☐	☐	☐				
GvHD related lesions of GIT	☐	☐	☐				
hepatic signs of GvHD	☐	☐	☐				
	☐	☐	☐				

*) In case there are signs and symptoms of GvHD please be sure to fill in the subsequent 2 sets of questions!

1. if appropriate please specify:

Karnofsky score at diagnosis of chronic GvHD [%] - see Annex 8.4	

2. diagnosis based on:

histological signs please specify	
clinical symptoms, please specify	

7.11 Specific Therapy for GvHD

yes ☐, no ☐, unknown ☐, if yes please be sure to enter the data required in table 4.4. The appropriate form of entry applies to this type of therapy also.

8.1   IAEA International nuclear event scale

Level	Descriptor	Criteria	Examples
Accidents			
7	Major Accident	• External release of a large fraction of the reactor core inventory typically involving a mixture of short and long-lived radioactive fission products (in quantities radiologically equivalent to more than tens of thousands TBq of ^{131}J). • Possibility of acute health effects. Delayed health effects over a wide area, possibly involving more than one country. Long term environmental consequences.	Chernobyl, SU, 1986
6	Serious Accident	• External release of fission products (in quantities radiologically equivalent to the order of thousands to tens of thousands TBq of ^{131}J). Full implementation of local emergency plans most likely needed to limit serious health effects.	
5	Accident with off-site Risks	• External release of fission products (in quantities radiologically equivalent to the order of hundreds to of thousands TBq of ^{131}J). Partial implementation of emergency plans (e. g., local sheltering and/or evacuation) required in some cases to lessen the likelihood of health effects. • Severe damage to large fraction of the core due to mechanical effects and/or melting.	Windscale, UK, 1957 Three Mile Island, USA, 1979
4	Accident Mainly in Installation	• External release of radioactivity, resulting in a dose to the most exposed individual off-site of the order of a few mSv. Need for off-site protective actions generally unlikely except possibly for local food control. • Some damage to reactor core due to mechanical effects and/or melting. • Worker doses that can lead to acute health effects (of the order of 1 Sv).	Saint Laurent, F, 1980
Incidents			
3	Serious Incident	• External release of radioactivity above authorised limits, resulting in a dose to the most exposed individual off-site of the order of tenths of a mSv. Off-site protective measures not needed. • High radiation levels and/or contamination on-site due to equipment failures or operational incidents. Overexposure of workers (individual doses exceeding 50 mSv). • Incidents in which a further failure of safety systems could lead to accident conditions, or a situation in which safety systems would be unable to prevent an accident if certain initiators were to occur.	Vandellos, E, 1989
2	Incident	• Technical incidents or anomalies which, although not directly or immediately affecting plant safety, are liable to lead to subsequent re-evaluation of safety provisions.	
1	Anomaly	• Functional or operational anomalies which do not pose a risk but which indicate a lack of safety provisions. This may be do to equipment failure, human error or procedural inadequacies. (Such anomalies should be distinguished from situations where operational limits and conditions are not exceeded and which are properly managed in accordance with adequate procedures. These are typically "below-scale".)	
Below Scale			
0	No Safety Significance		

8.2 Conversion of Non-SI to SI Units

$$1 \text{ Ci} = 3{,}7 \times 10^{10} \text{ Bq} = \mathbf{37 \text{ GBq}}$$

$$1 \text{ mCi} = \mathbf{37 \text{ MBq}}$$

$$1 \text{ } \mu\text{Ci} = \mathbf{37 \text{ kBq}}$$

$$1 \text{ nCi} = \mathbf{37 \text{ Bq}}$$

$$1 \text{ rem} = 10^{-2} \text{ Sv} = \mathbf{10 \text{ mSv}}$$

$$1 \text{ mrem} = \mathbf{10 \text{ } \mu\text{Sv}}$$

8.3 Orders of Magnitude

Power	Magnitude	Abbreviation	Entry Format	Power	Magnitude	Abbreviation	Entry Format
10^{12}	Tera	T	e12	10^{-3}	Milli	m	e-3
10^{9}	Giga	G	e9	10^{-6}	Micro	μ	e-6
10^{6}	Mega	M	e6	10^{-9}	Nano	n	e-9
10^{3}	Kilo	k	e3	10^{-12}	Piko	p	e-12

8.4 Karnofsky Scale for Rating Activity Status

Overall Rating	Percentage	Description
Able to carry on normal activity.	100	Normal; no complaints; no evidence of disease; no special care is needed
	90	Able to carry on normal activity.
	80	Normal activity with effort.
Unable to work; able to live at home, and take care of most personal needs; a varying amount of assistance is needed.	70	Cares for self; unable to carry out normal activities or to do active work.
	60	Requires occasional assistance but is able to take care of most needs.
	50	Requires considerable assistance and frequent medical care.
Unable to care for self; requires equivalent of institutional or hospital care; disease may be progressing rapidly.	40	Disabled; requires special care and assistance.
	30	Severely disabled; hospitalisation indicated, although death not imminent.
	20	Very sick; hospitalisation necessary.
	10	Moribund; fatal process progressing rapidly.
	0	Dead.

8.5 References

(the source material where the data of this questionnaire are taken from)

8.6   Normal Values of Laboratory Parameters

You are kindly requested to enter the upper and lower borders of your laboratory values. Please feel free to give your comments, e. g., on the method used (for further explanation see examples in the introduction).

Parameter Name	Unit	Lower Border (- 2 x SD)	Upper Border (+ 2 x SD)	Comment
Peripheral Blood Count				
Red Blood Cells	[Tera/l]			
Haemoglobin	[g/l]			
Haematocrit	[%]			
Mean Corpuscular Volume (MCV)	[femto-l]			
Reticulocytes	[%]			
Platelets	[Giga/l]			
Erythrocyte Sedimentation Rate (ESR)	[mm/h]			
White Blood Cells (WBC)	[Giga/l]			
Granulocytes	[Giga/l]			
Lymphocytes	[Giga/l]			
Peripheral Blood Smear				
Metamyelocyte	[Giga/l]			
Band Neutrophil Granulocyte	[Giga/l]			
Segmented Neutrophil Granuloc.	[Giga/l]			
Lymphocyte	[Giga/l]			
Monocyte	[Giga/l]			
Plasmacells	[Giga/l]			
Basophils	[Giga/l]			
Eosinophils	[Giga/l]			
Blasts	[Giga/l]			
Myeloblasts	[Giga/l]			
Promyelocytes	[Giga/l]			
Myelocytes	[Giga/l]			

Parameter Name	Unit	Lower Border (- 2 x SD)	Upper Border (+ 2 x SD)	Comment
Mitotic Connected Anomalies of Red Blood Cells	[No./No. of WBC counted]			
Mit. Conn. Anom. of Granulocytes	[%]			
Mit. Conn. Anom. of Lymphocytes	[%]			
Gigantic Granulocytes	[%]			
Atypical / Unidentified	[No./No. of WBC counted]			
Bone Marrow Examination				
Myelopoietic Tissue	[%]			
No. of Nucleated Cells	[Giga/l]			
Mitotic Connected Anomalies of Erythropoiesis	[%]			
Mitotic Connected Anomalies of Myeolopoiesis	[%]			
Blast	[%]			
Myeloblast	[%]			
Promyelocyte	[%]			
Myelocyte	[%]			
Metamyelocyte	[%]			
Band Neutrophil Granulocyte	[%]			
Segmented Neutrophil Granulocyte	[%]			
Basophil	[%]			
Eosinophilic Myelocyte	[%]			
Eosinophilic Metamyelocyte	[%]			
Eosinophil	[%]			

Parameter Name	Unit	Lower Border (- 2 x SD)	Upper Border (+ 2 x SD)	Comment
Lymphocyte	[%]			
Monocyte	[%]			
Plasmacell	[%]			
Makrophages	[%]			
Normoblast Mitoses	[%]			
Erythroblast	[%]			
Basophilic Normoblast	[%]			
Polynormoblast	[%]			
Oxyphilic Normoblast	[%]			
Megakaryocyte	[%]			
Gigantic Neutrophil	[%]			
Degenerated Neutrophil	[%]			
Degenerated Neutrophil	[%]			
Jolly's Bodies	[%]			
Cytogenetic Data				
Number of Cells Scored				
No. of Cells with Chromosomal Aberration(s)				
No. of Cells with Chromatid Aberr.				
No. of Aberrant Cells				
Dicentrics				
Rings				
Acentrics				
Chromatide Breaks				
Chromatide Exchanges				

Parameter Name	Unit	Lower Border (- 2 x SD)	Upper Border (+ 2 x SD)	Comment
Sex Chromosomes XX/XY				
No. cells with Aneupleoidy				
Aneupleoidy No. of Chromosomes				
Atypical Chromosomes				
Biochemical Data				
Bilirubin, total	[µmol/l]			
Bilirubin, direct	[µmol/l]			
ALT	[U/l]			
AST	[U/l]			
γ-GT	[U/l]			
LDH (total)	[U/l]			
LDH-I	[U/l]			
LDH-II	[U/l]			
LDH-III	[U/l]			
LDH-IV	[U/l]			
LDH-V	[U/l]			
Acetylcholineste-rase	[U/l]			
Alkaline Phosphatase	[U/l]			
CK	[U/l]			
CK-MB	[U/l]			
Amylase in Serum	[U/l]			
Cholesterol	[mmol/l]			
Urea	[mmol/l]			

Parameter Name	Unit	Lower Border (- 2 x SD)	Upper Border (+ 2 x SD)	Comment
Uric Acid	[μmol/l]			
Glucose in Serum	[mmol/l]			
Creatinine	[μmol/l]			
Total Protein	[g/l]			
Albumin	[g/l]			
α1-Globulin	[g/l]			
α2-Globulin	[g/l]			
β-Globulin	[g/l]			
γ-Globulin	[g/l]			
K	[mmol/l]			
Na	[mmol/l]			
Ca	[mmol/l]			
Fe	[μmol/l]			
Serum-Phosphorus	[mmol/l]			
Chloride	[mmol/l]			
Haemostatic Parameters				
PTT	[s]			
PT (QUICK)	[%]			
TT	[s]			
Fibrinogen	[μmol/l]			
Ethanol-Test	scores [0-4]			

Parameter Name	Unit	Lower Border (- 2 x SD)	Upper Border (+ 2 x SD)	Comment
Protamin Sulphate Test	scores [0-4]			
Retraction-Test	[0.0 - 1.0]			
Bleeding-Time DUKE	[min]			
Factor II	[%]			
Factor V	[%]			
Factor VIII	[%]			
Factor IX	[%]			
Factor X	[%]			
Fibrinolytic Activity	[min]			
Antithrombin III	[U/l]			
Immunological Parameters				
C-Reactive Protein	[g/l]			
T-Cells	[%]			
T-Helper	[%]			
T-Suppresser	[%]			
B-Cells	[%]			
IgG	[g/l]			
IgA	[g/l]			
IgM	[g/l]			
Complement	[g/l]			

Parameter Name	Unit	Lower Border (- 2 x SD)	Upper Border (+ 2 x SD)	Comment
Immunohaema-tological Tests				
Isohaemag-glutinin α	[1:n]			
Isohaemag-glutinin β	[1:n]			

Parameter Name	Unit	Lower Border (- 2 x SD)	Upper Border (+ 2 x SD)	Comment
Thyroid Hormones				
TSH	[mU/l]			
T3	[μmol/l]			
T4	[μmol/l]			
Blood Gas Analysis				
pO₂	[mm Hg]			
pCO₂	[mm Hg]			
pH	[]			
Base Excess	[mmol/l]			
Base-Buffer	[mmol/l]			
Hb-O₂	[%]			
Acid Buffer	[mmol/l]			
SBC	[%]			
--HCO₃	[mmol/l]			
Urine				
Glucose	[mmol/l]			
Uric Acid	[mmol/l]			
Creatinine	[mmol/l]			
Total Protein	[g/l]			
Albumin	[g/l]			
Amylase in Urine	[U/l]			
Na	[mmol/l]			

Parameter Name	Unit	Lower Border (- 2 x SD)	Upper Border (+ 2 x SD)	Comment
K	[mmol/l]			
Ca	[mmol/l]			
Chloride	[mmol/l]			
Urine-Phosphorus	[mmol/l]			
Specific Gravity	[#]			
Osmolarity	[mOsm/l]			
pH	[#]			
Amount of Urine per day	[l/d]			
WBC per Field	[#]			
RBC per Field	[#]			
Casts per Field	[#]			

8.7 Pages for copying

8.7.1 Symptoms and Signs

Symptom/Sign	yes	no	uk	Begin (Date & Time)	End (Date & Time)	Maximum (Date & Time)	Degree
	☐	☐	☐				
	☐	☐	☐				
	☐	☐	☐				
	☐	☐	☐				
	☐	☐	☐				
	☐	☐	☐				
	☐	☐	☐				
	☐	☐	☐				
	☐	☐	☐				
	☐	☐	☐				
	☐	☐	☐				
	☐	☐	☐				

8.7.2   Laboratory Values (left & right)

	Date and Time								
1									
2									
3									
4									
5									
6									
7									
8									
9									
10									
11									
12									
13									
14									
15									
16									
17									
18									
19									
20									
21									
22									
23									
24									
25									
26									
27									
28									
29									
30									

1											
2											
3											
4											
5											
6											
7											
8											
9											
10											
11											
12											
13											
14											
15											
16											
17											
18											
19											
20											
21											
22											
23											
24											
25											
26											
27											
28											
29											
30											

8.7.3   Normal Values

Parameter Name	Unit	Lower Border (- 2 x SD)	Upper Border (+ 2 x SD)	Comment

8.7.4   Antibiogramm (left) [†]

Date and Time				
Source of Material				
Species				
No. of Microbes per g or ml of Material				
Drugs :				
1				
2				
3				
4				
5				
6				
7				
8				
9				
10				
11				
12				
13				
14				
15				
16				
17				
18				
19				
20				
21				
22				
23				
24				
25				
26				
27				
28				
29				
30				
31				
32				
33				

[†] Please indicate the degree of sensitivity as follows:

very sensitive   +   sensitive   o   not sensitive   -   unknown or not tested   uk

8.7.5 Antibiogramm (right) ✝

1					
2					
3					
4					
5					
6					
7					
8					
9					
10					
11					
12					
13					
14					
15					
16					
17					
18					
19					
20					
21					
22					
23					
24					
25					
26					
27					
28					
29					
30					
31					
32					
33					

✝ Please indicate the degree of sensitivity as follows: